Springer

Tokyo
Berlin
Heidelberg
New York
Barcelona
Hong Kong
London
Milan
Paris
Singapore

K. Okita (Ed.)

HCV and Related Liver Diseases

With 23 Figures

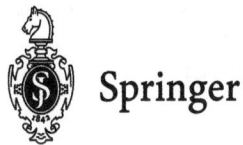 Springer

KIWAMU OKITA, M.D., Ph.D.
Professor and Chairman,
First Department of Internal Medicine,
Yamaguchi University School of Medicine
Kogushi, Ube, Yamaguchi, 755-8505, JAPAN

ISBN-13: 978-4-431-68490-9   e-ISBN-13: 978-4-431-68488-6
DOI: 10.1007/ 978-4-431-68488-6

Printed on acid-free paper

© Springer-Verlag Tokyo 1999
Softcover reprint of the hardcover 1st edition

Typesetting, printing, and binding: Best-set Typesetter Ltd., Hong Kong

SPIN: 10681426

Preface

The ninth meeting of the Yamaguchi Symposium on Liver Disease, held every December since its inception in 1986, convened December 13–14, 1997.

With astonishing progress in recent research on viral hepatitis, it seemed the time to summarize and present the work that had been done to date. Therefore, at the recommendation of Emeritus Professor Fumihiro Ichida, a pioneer in hepatitis research in Japan, and members of the Organizing Committee, viral hepatitis was chosen as the main theme for the symposium.

It is estimated that more than 2 million people in Japan have the hepatitis C virus (HCV). Of these, 300000 will die of liver cirrhosis and another 30000 will lose their lives as a result of complications of hepatocellular carcinoma. Although the information has not been verified, in the United States the number of persons with liver disease caused by HCV is said to be approaching 4 million. Therefore, much more attention must be given to HCV-related liver diseases while continuing to be concerned with diseases caused by hepatitis B virus (HBV).

Leading Japanese hepatologists were invited to the ninth symposium, where they took part in serious discussions of the following major topics: (1) Possible replication of HCV in peripheral blood mononuclear cells; (2) Clinical manifestations other than liver disease in patients who are HCV-positive; (3) Biological characteristics of HCV; (4) More effective treatment of chronic hepatitis C, particularly with a combination of different antiviral agents; (5) The possible chemoprevention by interferon of hepatocellular carcinoma.

We were fortunate that Professor Stanley M. Lemon was able to accept our invitation to the symposium. Prof. Lemon is one of the top virologists and hepatologists and on the American side is in charge of the U.S.–Japan Hepatitis Conference. His remarks on the virological aspects of HCV were extremely valuable to participants concerned with treatment of chronic hepatitis C.

Two days of discussions made clear that we do not yet have extremely effective antiviral agents for chronic hepatitis C, nor is there evidence that HCV behaves like an oncogenic virus, in spite of a positive epidemiological relationship between HCV and hepatocellular carcinoma. In dealing with HCV infection and disease, much work remains to be done in developing more effective therapies to reduce the number of patients who are at risk of dying of advanced chronic liver diseases.

The symposium could not have been held without the generous financial support of the Otsuka Pharmaceutical Co., Ltd., to whom the Organizing Committee, on behalf of all participants, expresses sincere gratitude for their continuing, valuable assistance.

Finally, The Organizing Committee sincerely hopes that this proceedings, with its wealth of information, is useful for physicians and hepatologists around the world who are involved in this specific field.

ORGANIZING COMMITTEE OF THE YAMAGUCHI SYMPOSIUM
ON LIVER DISEASE
Kiwamu Okita, M.D., Yamaguchi University, Ube
Kenichi Kobayashi, M.D., Kanazawa University, Kanazawa
Masamichi Kojiro, M.D., Kurume University, Kurume
Masao Omata, M.D., University of Tokyo, Tokyo

Table of Contents

List of Participants

Fukumoto, Yohei	Department of General Internal Medicine Yamaguchi University School of Medicine Yamaguchi, Japan
Hayashi, Norio	First Department of Medicine Osaka University School of Medicine Osaka, Japan
Hino, Keisuke	First Department of Internal Medicine Yamaguchi University School of Medicine Yamaguchi, Japan
Honda, Masao	First Department of Internal Medicine Kanazawa University School of Medicine Ishikawa, Japan
Ichida, Fumihiro	Professor Emeritus Niigata University School of Medicine Niigata, Japan
Ichida, Takafumi	Third Department of Medicine Niigata University School of Medicine Niigata, Japan
Kakumu, Shinichi	First Department of Internal Medicine Aichi Medical University Aichi, Japan
Kasahara, Akinori	First Department of Medicine Osaka University School of Medicine Osaka, Japan
Kato, Naoya	Second Department of Internal Medicine University of Tokyo School of Medicine Tokyo, Japan

Kobayashi, Kenichi	First Department of Internal Medicine Kanazawa University School of Medicine Ishikawa, Japan
Kojiro, Masamichi	First Department of Pathology Kurume University School of Medicine Fukuoka, Japan
Lemon, Stanley M.	Department of Microbiology and Immunology The University of Texas Medical Branch at Galveston Texas, U.S.A.
Mizokami, Masashi	Second Department of Medicine Nagoya City University Medical School Nagoya, Japan
Nakanishi, Toshio	First Department of Medicine Hiroshima University School of Medicine Hiroshima, Japan
Nakano, Tatsunori	Second Department of Medicine Nagoya City University Medical School Nagoya, Japan
Nishiguchi, Shuhei	Third Department of Medicine Osaka City University School of Medicine Osaka, Japan
Okita, Kiwamu	First Department of Internal Medicine Yamaguchi University School of Medicine Yamaguchi, Japan
Omata, Masao	Second Department of Internal Medicine University of Tokyo School of Medicine Tokyo, Japan
Orito, Etsuro	Second Department of Medicine Nagoya City University Medical School Nagoya, Japan
Sakaida, Isao	First Department of Internal Medicine Yamaguchi University School of Medicine Yamaguchi, Japan

Sata, Michio   Second Department of Medicine
                      Kurume University School of Medicine
                      Fukuoka, Japan

Tanikawa, Kyuichi   Second Department of Medicine
                      Kurume University School of Medicine
                      Fukuoka, Japan

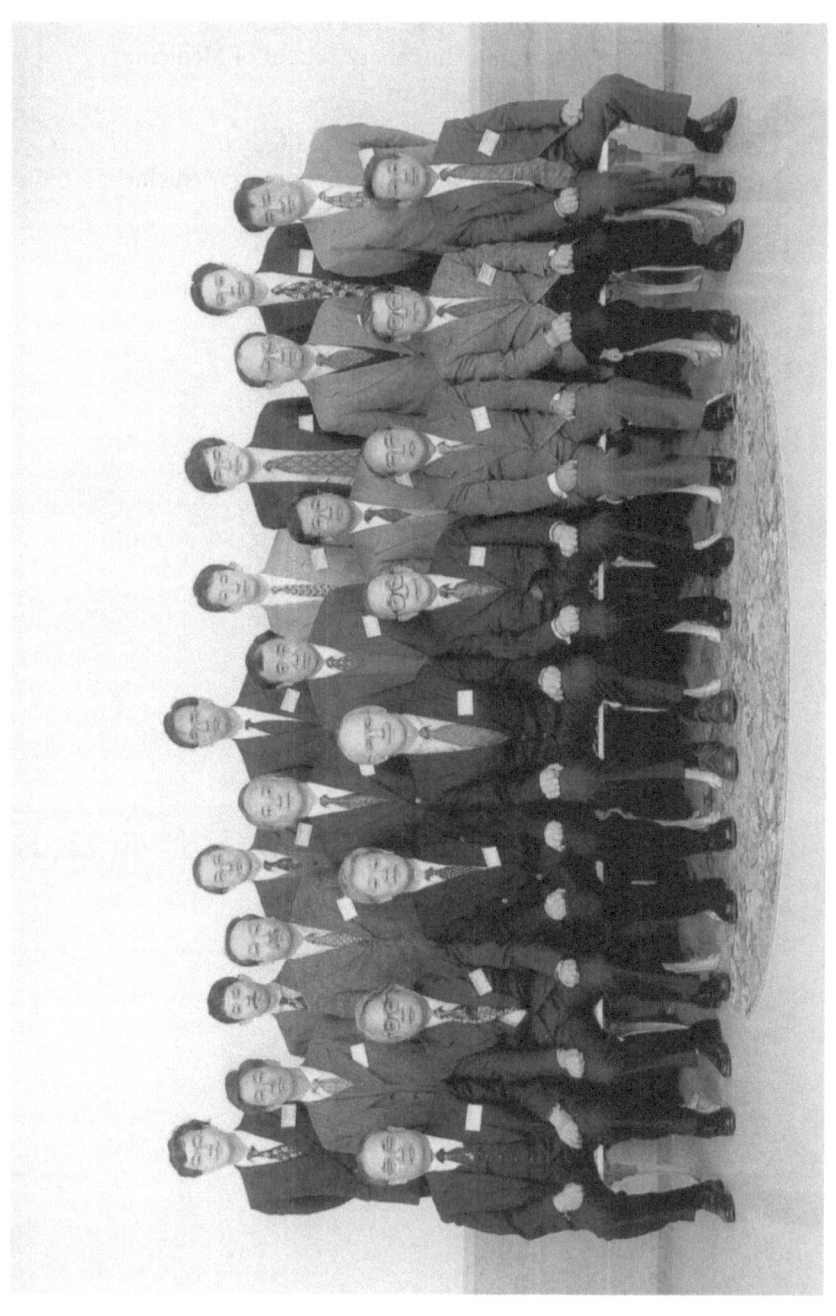

Hepatitis C: Current Status and Future Directions for Antiviral Therapy

STANLEY M. LEMON

Introduction

Hepatitis C virus (HCV) was first identified and shown to be the cause of almost all cases of non-B posttransfusion hepatitis in the late 1980s [1,2]. The virus, now classified within the genus Hepacivirus of the family Flaviviridae, is unique in its ability to establish persistent infection in the great majority of infected persons, many of whom develop evidence of chronic inflammatory liver disease [3]. These chronically infected persons are at risk for cirrhosis and, to a lesser extent, hepatocellular carcinoma [4,5]. Such serious complications of HCV infection usually develop over several decades, although in exceptional cases life-threatening liver disease can become evident within 10 years or less of infection. Despite this, most infected individuals appear to reach a relatively healthy equilibrium with this infection, and the majority of infected persons will probably die of causes completely unrelated to hepatitis C. Little is known of the reasons why certain infected patients do well, while others get into trouble with this infection. This lack of understanding extends to an absence of prognostic tests that are capable of predicting disease outcome in individual patients.

Another unexplained mystery is that most American patients who do succumb to liver disease related to chronic hepatitis C die as a result of cirrhosis and liver failure, while most HCV-related deaths in Japan are due to hepatocellular carcinoma [6]. The factors that may account for this apparent difference in the natural history of the infection are not known. However, these may include genetic differences in the populations of the two countries, dietary or other environmental factors, differences in the

Department of Microbiology and Immunology, The University of Texas Medical Branch at Galveston, Galveston, TX 77555-1019, USA infecting strains of HCV, differences in the age-specific distribution of HCV infections in the two countries, or other yet unrecognized factors.

Epidemiology of Hepatitis C: Contrasting Patterns in the US and Japan

HCV infection accounts for under 20% of acute viral hepatitis cases within the United States. However, it is by far the leading cause of chronic viral hepatitis and is present in 40%–55% of persons who succumb to chronic liver disease of any type. The Centers for Disease Control and Prevention (Atlanta, GA, USA) recently estimated that HCV infection contributes to as many as 8000–10000 deaths annually due to chronic liver disease within the United States [7]. A recent serologic survey of over 20000 Americans has been carried out by this government agency using sera that were collected by a stratified, randomized sampling of the population. The results of this study indicate that, overall, approximately 1.8% of all Americans are positive for HCV antibody, and thus most likely persistently infected with the virus. Strikingly higher prevalences of infection were documented in African Americans and Mexican Americans, compared with Caucasian Americans. Most importantly, the highest prevalences of infection were noted in persons aged 30 to 50 years, with substantially lower antibody prevalences found in older persons of any racial background.

This pattern of the age-related seroprevalence of HCV infection strongly suggests that there has been an upsurge in new HCV infections among young adults over the past 2–3 decades. This is almost certainly related to increases in illicit injection drug use in the US since the early 1960s. Since HCV infection persists for many decades and progresses only slowly to serious liver disease, it is likely that this relatively recent epidemic spread of HCV will be reflected in substantial increases in liver-specific mortality during the next two decades. By the year 2010, it is predicted that the number of HCV-related deaths will increase to 24000–30000 per year [8]. This would represent a tripling of the present estimated death rate due to hepatitis C, and an annual HCV-related death rate comparable to the present number of AIDS-related deaths in the US.

These predictions are made credible by increases in the death rate due to HCV-associated hepatocellular carcinoma that have been observed over the past 20 years in Japan [9,10]. During this period, the rate of death due to liver cancer tripled among Japanese men, and this increase in cancer deaths was related exclusively to HCV-associated tumors. Interestingly, there has been little increase in the incidence of liver tumors among Japanese women during the same period, despite the fact that the seroprevalence of HCV is roughly similar in both genders. Equally striking, however, is the age-related seroprevalence curve in Japan [11]. In contrast to the US, where a major peak is present in the 30–50-year-old age group, seroprevalence increases continuously with advancing age in Japan. This reflects the widespread dissemination of HCV infection within the Japanese population in the early post-WWII era, probably due to a combination of injection needle practices and frequent blood transfusions related to endemic tuberculosis.

Thus, both countries have experienced a cohort-effect with respect to HCV infection and disease during the last half of this century, with the Japanese experience preceding the American experience by 2–3 decades. This epidemiologic view is supported by phylogenetic analyses of HCV strains in the two countries, and is very sobering from the American perspective. It accentuates the need for a better understanding of the pathobiology of this infection, and the accelerated development of better therapies.

Mechanisms of HCV Replication: Ample Targets for Novel Antivirals

The HCV Polyprotein

Like other flaviviruses, HCV is a positive-strand RNA virus [12,13]. The virus particles possess an extensively glycosylated envelope within which the 9.7 kb single-stranded RNA genome is packaged in association with a highly basic, nucleocapsid (core) protein. As with many other positive-strand viruses, HCV expresses its protein complement in the form of a single giant polyprotein that is encoded by a large open reading frame extending through much of the length of the genomic RNA (Fig. 1). Unlike yellow fever virus and other members of the genus Flavivirus, HCV and other Flaviviridae classified with the genus Pestivirus initiate translation of this polyprotein via internal entry of the 40S ribosome subunit on the virion RNA. This process is controlled by a highly structured RNA sequence located within the 342 nucleotide-long 5' non-translated RNA (NTR), which is called the internal ribosome entry site (or IRES) [14]. The precise structure of the 5' end of the genomic RNA is not known, although it is presumed not to possess a typical 5' cap structure.

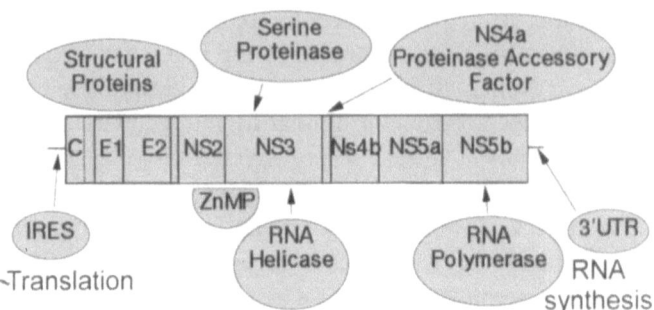

Fig. 1. Diagram depicting the genetic organization of the hepatitis C virus (HCV) genome. Major protein products derived from proteolytic processing of the polyprotein are indicated. *E1* and *E2*, secreted glycoproteins that form the envelope of the virus

The 3′ nontranslated RNA appears also to be relatively structured [15,16], but it also contains a lengthy pyrimidine-rich tract that is largely poly-(U) in composition. The function of this tract is unknown.

The polyprotein of HCV is comprised of approximately 3000 amino acid residues. It undergoes cotranslational and posttranslational cleavages that are directed by both host cell and virus-encoded proteinases (Fig. 1) [17–19]. Signal sequences located within the amino terminal third of the polyprotein direct its secretion into the endoplasmic reticulum (ER). There, several cleavages directed by host cell signalase produce a series of structural proteins. These include the nucleocapsid protein (otherwise known as the core protein), two envelope glycoproteins, E1 and E2, and a small membrane-associated protein, p7 (or NS2A) that plays an uncertain role in viral assembly. The nucleocapsid protein remains within the cytoplasm and may possibly undergo further proteolytic processing. In contrast, E1 and E2 are secreted, and extensively glycosylated within the ER and Golgi [20,21]. Their subsequent trafficking within the cell remains uncertain. However, there is little evidence that these glycoproteins reach the cell surface, and it is possible that viral assembly involves budding of virus particles into internal membranous structures within the cell.

The remaining segment of the polyprotein is processed entirely under the control of two viral proteinases. What may be a primary cleavage occurs at the NS2/NS3 junction, under control of a *cis*-acting zinc-dependent metalloproteinase that spans this junction [18,19]. Further processing of the polyprotein is controlled by the viral serine proteinase located within the amino terminal third of the NS3 protein, and is likely to involve both *cis*- and *trans*-active cleavages. A small polypeptide, NS4A, which appears to be cleaved from the residual amino end of the nascent polypeptide following the release of NS3, assembles noncovalently with the NS3 molecule to form a fully active proteinase [22,23]. Although the temporal sequence of the processing cascade remains poorly documented, this NS3/NS4A complex cleaves at several different sites within the polyprotein, resulting in several additional proteins (NS4B, NS5A, NS5B). While NS5B is an RNA-dependent RNA polymerase, the functional roles of these additional proteins are not well understood. Nonetheless, it is likely that each of the resulting cleavage products has a specific function related to replication of the RNA. In addition to its proteinase activities, NS3 has NTPase and RNA helicase activities mapping to its carboxy two-thirds [24,25]. NS4A plays a role in controlling the phosphorylation of NS5A [26], although the function of the latter protein remains uncertain.

Molecular Events in HCV Replication

Replication of the viral RNA proceeds through a negative-strand intermediate, and is likely to occur in association with membranous replication complexes in the cellular cytoplasm. These complexes almost certainly include each of the nonstructural proteins of the virus [27]. Initiation of negative-strand synthesis is likely to be dependent upon specific recognition of the 3'NTR RNA structure by this replicase complex. Among the HCV proteins, RNA binding activities are present within the core protein as well as NS3 and NS5B.

Similarly, the initiation of positive-strand RNA synthesis from newly synthesized negative-stranded RNA is also likely to require specific recognition of the 3' terminal negative-strand structure by the RNA replicase. This latter structure is of course formed by sequence complementary to the 5'NTR of the virion RNA. The extent to which recognition of the 3' and 5' ends of the RNA by the replicase complex include common RNA-binding activities is not known. However, it is noteworthy that there is no recognizable structural homology between the 3' ends of these RNA molecules. Replication of the RNAs appears to occur asymmetrically, with positive-strand synthesis exceeding negative-strand synthesis.

Remarkably, however, most studies indicate that infected liver contains less than 10-fold more copies of the positive-strand than the negative-strand [28]. This is very different from the situation with the picornavirus, hepatitis A virus (HAV), where the abundance of positive-strand copies exceeds the negative-strand intermediate by a factor of 100 or more [29].

Thus, although HCV is a relatively simple virus that expresses less than a dozen separate proteins, its replication is dependent upon a considerable number of virus-specified enzymatic activities or highly specific macromolecular interactions. Each of these is a potential target for development of new antiviral drugs. It is remarkable that a such a large amount of information has been gathered concerning a number of these viral activities, despite the fact that the virus is unable to replicate with any degree of efficiency in cell culture.

Potential Mechanisms Underlying Viral Persistence

The morbidity and mortality associated with HCV infection is due largely to its unique propensity to cause persistent infection in most persons, a feature that distinguishes this virus from other known hepatitis viruses [3]. Persistent infections with hepatitis B virus (HBV), for example, generally occur only in individuals who are immunocompromised, or who are infected at birth, while truly persistent infections with HAV occur rarely if ever. In sharp contrast, recent data from a cohort of injection drug users that has been studied prospectively in Baltimore by Thomas and colleagues suggest that persistent infection develops in about 85% of adults who undergo acute HCV infection with seroconversion to the virus [6]. Although the specific mechanisms underlying the persistence of HCV are not known, the available evidence suggests several possibilities.

Regulated Replication of HCV

Among potential mechanisms contributing to viral persistence is the possibility that the replication of HCV may be specifically regulated by a mechanism that minimizes the expression of viral proteins. From a teleological point of view, this would offer several survival advantages to the virus. First, it would contribute to the lack of cytopathic effect that appears to mark this flavivirus relatively uniquely. Second, it could conceivably lower the profile of the infection as seen by the host immune system, rendering an infected cell less likely to be recognized by virus-specific cytotoxic T lymphocytes (CTLs). There is no solid evidence for specific regulation of the HCV replication cycle. However, the hepaciviruses differ significantly from the flaviviruses and pestiviruses (other members of the family Flaviviridae) in that they lack the capacity for vigorous replication such as that observed with yellow fever virus or bovine viral diarrhea virus both in animals and in cell culture. It is noteworthy that HCV titers in the blood are never very high, even during acute infections before the evolution of virus-suppressive CTLs, despite the fact that the liver contains an enormous mass of apparently permissive hepatocytes.

Furthermore, it is curious that, while HCV does apparently undergo replication in cultured lymphoblastoid cells, it never adapts to growth in these cells [30–32]. HAV readily adapts to growth in monkey kidney cells over the course of 10–20 consecutive passages [33]. However, there is no significant increase in the replicative capacity of HCV, even after continuous passage for up to a year in lymphoblastoid cells. The infectious titer of the virus present in harvests of these cells never exceeds $2-3\log_{10}$/ml. This is puzzling for a positive-strand RNA virus that is known to undergo relatively frequent mutation during the course of human infection [34]. These observations suggest an intrinsic restriction on replication of the virus, at least in these cells.

A possible molecular mechanism for such regulation of virus replication is suggested by studies of the HCV IRES. Several lines of evidence suggest that the 40S ribosome subunit forms an important primary contact with the viral RNA directly at the site of the initiator AUG codon at nt 343 of the genome [35–37]. There is no scanning of the ribosome subunit on the RNA prior to its being positioned over the initiator AUG. Interestingly, the initiator AUG is located within the single-stranded RNA segment of what appears to be a small stem-loop (Fig. 2) [35]. Preservation of this structure is not required for IRES activity in synthetic RNA transcripts, and mutations which enhance its stability have a notable negative effect on virus translation. Yet, this RNA structure appears to be present in all strains of HCV that have been studied to date. One possible explanation for these findings is that the stem-loop might act as a regulator of translation, were it the target site of a viral RNA-binding protein that was capable of stabilizing this RNA structure through a protein–RNA interaction [35]. If this were the case, the viral protein could effectively compete with the 40S ribosome subunit for the viral RNA, providing a convenient mechanism for autoregulation of viral gene expression

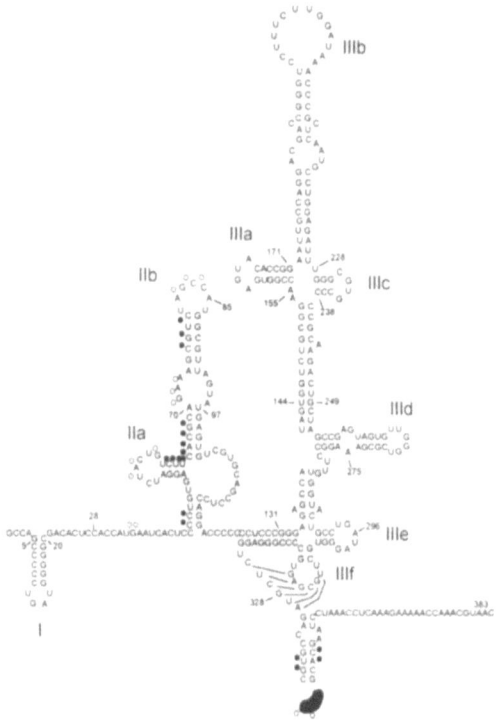

Fig. 2. Secondary and tertiary RNA structures that are present within the 5′ nontranslated RNA (5′NTR) of HCV and which control cap-independent translation of the virus by a process of internal ribosome entry. A primary contact is formed between the 40S subunit and the viral RNA near the site of the initiator AUG (*shaded box*), which is located within the single-stranded sequence of a small stem-loop [35]. Modified from Lemon and Honda [14]

through translational repression. There are as yet no hard data that support the autoregulation of HCV translation by an HCV gene product, but very similar regulatory mechanisms have been demonstrated to exist among some prokaryotic viruses.

Quasispecies Variation

Like the human immunodeficiency virus (HIV-1), HCV demonstrates extensive nucleotide sequence variation within individual patients. The virus is present in blood as a diversity of genetically related but individually distinct sequences (i.e., a quasispecies "swarm") [34]. The extent of quasispecies variation is dependent on two major factors: the extent of ongoing viral replication, and the presence of selective forces which favor the amplification of certain quasispecies over others. Viral replication is essential to this phenomenon, because it is the machine that allows the virus to explore "sequence space" (i.e., all possible virus sequences). The RNA polymerase, like all viral RNA-dependent RNA polymerases, lacks a proofreading capability and makes relatively frequent errors during RNA transcription. On average, this is likely to amount to more than one misincorporated base in every progeny RNA molecule. The primary selective forces that shape the process of quasispecies variation include the replication capacity of the variant RNA, and immunologic pressure applied by CTL activity and neutralizing antibodies. These latter forces lead to the continued evolution of both B- and T-cell escape mutants in chronically infected persons [38–40].

The role played by this quasispecies variation in the establishment of persistent infection has been extensively debated. Although genetic variation is extensive, it is far from clear that it is a cause of virus persistence. It seems more likely that quasispecies variation occurs as a result of persistence, with continuous replication providing the virus with the opportunity to explore sequence space. According to this hypothesis, the evolution of escape mutants is then a reflection of the presence of an active yet ultimately ineffective immune response to this infection.

Potential Role of the Envelope Glycosylation in Viral Persistence

The envelope proteins of HCV are glycosylated to an unusual extent, as the addition of microsomal membrane preparations to cell-free translation reactions results in an approximate doubling of the molecular masses of both E1 and E2 [17]. This is reminiscent of the extensive glycosylation of the envelope protein of HIV. The glycosylation of the HCV envelope proteins likely reduces the ability of the immune system to respond effectively to the presence of these proteins. On the whole, there is relatively little evidence for neutralizing antibodies that are capable of significantly reducing viral infectivity. The absence of an effective neutralizing antibody response is reflected in generally high levels of anti-E2 antibodies in individuals who are viremic with HCV [41]. Another measure of the lack of an effective neutralization response is the high frequency of second infections observed in chimpanzees on reexposure to an HCV inoculum that was previously used to infect the animal [42]. However, more detailed studies of the neutralizing antibody response to HCV are not possible due to the absence of an effective cell culture system for propagation of the virus. This has precluded the development of classical viral neutralization assays.

Despite these indications of a poor overall neutralizing antibody response to HCV, the E2 protein contains a highly variable domain near its amino terminus (HVR-1 domain). This domain appears to form an immunogenic loop on the surface of the virion and it is suspected to interact with neutralizing antibodies [38,43]. The HVR-1 domain is a prime site for the evolution of quasispecies mutations. What specific role it might play in the pathobiology of this infection is unclear.

Could HCV Specifically Disarm the Immune System?

Despite the above speculations, it seems likely that HCV, like many other viruses, may have evolved specific mechanisms for evasion of the host immune system. There are two suggestive lines of evidence for this. First, the core protein of HCV has been shown to interact directly with the cytoplasmic domain of the lymphocytotoxin beta receptor and other members of the tumor necrosis factor (TNF) receptor family [44]. The evidence suggests that this interaction occurs close to the "death domain" through which an apoptotic signal is transduced to the nucleus following the binding of ligand to the receptor. Although the molecular evidence for this interaction is strong, its biologic significance remains uncertain. Initially suspected of potentially blocking signal transduction (and thereby protecting the infected cell from attack by CTLs), recent evidence suggests that the expression of core protein may actually sensitize some cells to apoptosis following the binding of ligand [45–47]. While this makes little sense in the context of infected hepatocytes, there is evidence that suggests that HCV may also infect lymphoid cells [31,48]. In this case, early apoptosis may prevent an infected lymphoid cell from participating in the activation of CTLs or the production of antibody. Clearly, more work is needed in this area, but efforts will be slowed by the continued absence of a small animal model for hepatitis C.

A second possible way in which HCV could interfere with the host immune response concerns the cellular interferon-inducible kinase, PKR. Phosphorylation of this kinase is induced by the presence of double-stranded RNA, and phosphorylated PKR acts to inhibit host cell translation through phosphorylation of the cellular translation initiation factor, eIF-2. This results in both an antiviral and antiproliferative state in the cell. Following discovery of an "interferon sensitivity determining region" (ISDR) within the NS5A protein [49,50], it was shown recently that NS5A interacts directly with the catalytic domain of PKR [51]. This suggests that the presence of NS5A might create a cellular environment within which interferon-mediated antiviral responses are relatively ineffectual. This is an attractive hypothesis, because the virus clearly is able to survive the endogenous host interferon response, despite its suppression by exogenous interferon administered in large doses. However, as with the core–TNF receptor interaction, the biologic significance of the NS5A-PKR interaction remains to be proven.

Careful consideration of the mechanisms underlying viral persistence will be important to gaining an understanding of the pathobiology of hepatitis C. It may even lead to novel strategies for intervention. However, it is important to remember that there may be no single underlying cause for HCV persistence. Instead, persistent infections may result from a combination of factors, including both those that are described above as well as others that are waiting to be discovered.

Vaccines Versus Antiviral Agents in the Control of Hepatitis C

In addition to quasispecies variation, there is considerable genetic diversity among different strains of HCV [34]. Although classical neutralization assays have not been developed and data are thus sparse, it is likely that these different HCV genotypes also vary substantially in their antigenicity. Pairwise comparisons of the nucleotide sequences of NS5B from different HCV genotypes reveal a magnitude of difference that is far greater than that which exists between the RNA polymerase (3Dpol) sequences of types 1 and 2 poliovirus. This suggests that different HCV genotypes may well be different serotypes in that they may stimulate little if any cross-protective immunity to each other. However, as indicated above, we lack the tools (neutralization assays and small animal models) that would be required to test this point.

Thus, genetic, and likely antigenic, variation poses major problems for the development of vaccines against HCV. To a large extent, the technical hurdles in HCV vaccine development mirror those that have been encountered in HIV vaccine development. Although a candidate vaccine comprised of recombinant envelope proteins was shown to protect chimpanzees against a low-dose homologous challenge [52], the ability of such a vaccine to protect against other HCV strains is doubtful at best. It is an important point to test, however, and it would be premature to consider dropping such a conventional approach to vaccine development. In the long run, however, it seems likely that the extent of antigenic variation among the envelope glycoproteins may ultimately point this field in the direction of T cell vaccines. Such a vaccine has been shown capable of protecting mice from infection with lymphocytic chorio-meningitis virus [53].

In the absence of any clearly feasible strategy that might allow development of effective immunization against hepatitis C, only three general approaches offer any hope of decreasing the disease burden due to HCV infection. First, new infections may be prevented in the absence of effective vaccines by screening blood products that pose risks for transmission of HCV. Although it is likely that a small number of transfusion-related cases of hepatitis C continue to occur, this approach has been spectacularly successful in reducing the frequency of transfusion-related hepatitis C since 1991 in many countries [7,54,55]. However, the impact of blood screening is of course limited by the extent to which other mechanisms of transmission (e.g., injection drug use) contribute proportionately to new infections.

A second approach is to foster modification of risky behaviors in certain high-risk populations (i.e., injection drug users). This may be more difficult to achieve than screening the blood supply. However, there have been significant decreases in the incidence of all forms of viral hepatitis associated with illicit injection drug use within the United States over the past decade. The basis for these decreases is far from clear, but it is likely that they reflect a reduction in risky needle-sharing behaviors related to the fear of AIDS. Whatever the reason, there has been a dramatic decrease in the incidence of new HCV infections within the United States since 1988 [7]. Nonetheless, approximately 4 million persons remain persistently infected with HCV within the United States alone. These individuals, most of whom are currently in their third and fourth decades of life as indicated above, will remain at significant risk for cirrhosis and hepatocellular carcinoma in the absence of new therapeutic modalities.

The third and last general strategy is the development of better therapeutic regimens that are capable of reducing or possibly even eliminating the liver destructive effects of HCV infection.

Interferon Treatment of Chronic Hepatitis C

A considerable number of controlled clinical trials have proven that treatment with several different formulations of interferon may be beneficial in a small proportion of patients with chronic hepatitis C [8]. This beneficial response is marked by normalization of serum alanine aminotransferase (ALT) values, elimination of viral RNA, and/or improvements in hepatic histology. A full discussion of these reports is well beyond the scope of this review. However, several points are worth emphasizing. First of all, the mechanism by which interferon exerts its therapeutic benefit is not well understood. There is a clear antiviral effect, with relatively rapid declines in HCV viremia on institution of interferon therapy. However, it is not clear whether this reflects a direct suppression of viral replication, or enhanced immunologic suppression of viral replication due to the immunomodulatory action of interferon. The latter includes the up-regulation of class I markers on the surface of hepatocytes, which would enhance the recognition of infected cells by virus-specific CTLs.

It is interesting to note, however, that improved liver histology is the measure of response to interferon that occurs with the greatest frequency in treated patients. This significantly exceeds the frequency with which ALT levels are normalized or viral RNA eliminated. In early randomized, placebo-controlled, prospective clinical trials, improvements in histology occurred in an average of about 70% of all patients with hepatitis C who were treated with interferon [56–58]. In contrast, ALT levels became normal in only about 40% of patients by the end of 6 months of therapy with 2–3 million units interferon-α thrice per week. Thus, whatever the underlying therapeutic mechanism, at least a transient reduction in hepatic inflammation frequently accompanies interferon therapy.

This suggests that interferon may have a significant impact on the outcome of the disease, but data supporting a tangible improvement in health or quality of life have been sparse. Nonetheless, one randomized, controlled, prospective study has demonstrated a reduction in the incidence of hepatocellular carcinoma in Japanese patients with well compensated cirrhosis who were given relatively high-dose interferon therapy (6 million units of interferon-α three times a week for 12–24 weeks) [59]. Hepatologists in the west have been slow to accept these results due to the extraordinarily high incidence of liver cancer that was reported in the control group in this study. This approached 40% after 2–7 years of posttreatment follow-up. However, it is likely that the high incidence of cancer in the untreated patients may simply reflect the natural history of hepatitis C in Japan, which appears to differ from that in the US as indicated above [6,60]. At least two additional, retrospective studies (one in Japan and one in Europe) suggest similar conclusions [61]. These studies, one of which was presented at this symposium, suggest that patients who respond to interferon have a lower risk of developing hepatocellular carcinoma than interferon nonresponders.

In addition to a relatively low response rate, there are other major impediments to successful treatment of chronic hepatitis C with interferon. These include the extraordinarily high cost of the drug, its administration, and attendant patient monitoring. Moreover, interferon therapy for chronic hepatitis C is marked by a relatively high frequency of adverse side effects such as cytopenia, depression, autoimmunity, and increased frequency of bacterial infections, among others. Most notable, however, is the high rate of relapse that typically follows completion of interferon therapy. This generally occurs in about half of all treated patients whose ALT levels have been rendered normal by the end of therapy, although it may occur in a slightly smaller proportion of patients if therapy is continued for a year [8]. The low overall frequency of sustained response to interferon is a major reason for the current intensive search for better therapeutic regimens.

Approach to Antiviral Therapy—The Case for Combination Therapy

Recent successes in the treatment of HIV-1 infections with combinations of antiviral drugs argue strongly for a similar approach to the treatment of chronic HCV infection. This is particularly so since HCV infections share a number of features in common with persistent HIV-1 infection, including the capacity for substantial quasispecies variation and the potential for selection of resistant viruses in patients receiving monotherapy. Combination therapy with antimicrobial agents has a long history in the treatment of chronic infectious diseases. It has been used for decades in the treatment of tuberculosis for very similar reasons. In the case of hepatitis C, recent data strongly support a synergistic effect when ribavirin is combined with interferon, both in interferon-naïve patients as well as in the retreatment of interferon nonresponders.

Ribavirin is a synthetic, oral guanosine nucleoside analog that has been used clinically for a number of years as treatment for several different viral infections. It has demonstrated efficacy in the treatment of neonatal respiratory syncytial virus infections, as well as in life-threatening arenavirus infections [62,63]. The compound is unusual in that it possesses a broad range of antiviral activity against viruses of vastly different type. It has been suggested to block the synthesis of functional rhabdovirus mRNAs [64], possibly by interfering with capping of the 5′ ends of the RNA (a phenomenon that is likely to be irrelevant in the case of HCV). Other data suggest that it may suppress transcription of double-stranded reovirus RNAs, possibly by interfering with viral RNA helicase activity [65]. However, its mode of broad antiviral action has never been satisfactorily explained and, as indicated below, it may have important immunomodulatory activities.

Early studies of ribavirin monotherapy in patients with chronic hepatitis C were prompted by its known activity against other RNA virus infections. For the most part, these studies were disappointing. Although slow improvement was noted in serum ALT values, there was very little suppression of HCV viremia even after prolonged therapy. This indicates that the antiviral effect of ribavirin against HCV, if any, is extremely limited [66–69].

Despite the early results with ribavirin monotherapy, recent clinical trials indicate that the addition of ribavirin to standard courses of interferon results in significant increases in the response to therapy. This is marked by increases both in the proportion of patients with end-of-treatment responses, as well as in the proportion of patients with sustained responses. For example, in a prospective randomized trial, Lai et al. [70] treated interferon-naïve patients with the combination of ribavirin (1200 mg four times daily) and interferon-α 2a (3 million units thrice weekly) for 24 weeks. This combination treatment regimen resulted in a complete response (normalization of ALT and elimination of detectable HCV RNA) in 76% of patients by the end of therapy, and a sustained response at 96 weeks after therapy in 43% (Fig. 3). In contrast, comparable response rates in patients receiving a similar course of interferon without ribavirin were 32% and 6%, respectively.

Similar findings were reported recently by Reichard et al. [71] in a larger prospective study examining the combination of ribavirin and interferon-α 2b (3 million units thrice weekly), given for a total of 24 weeks. Altogether, 42% of the patients had a sustained virologic response after 1 year of follow-up, compared to only 20% of patients receiving interferon alone. Importantly, a retrospective analysis of the patients included in this study indicated that the combination was beneficial only

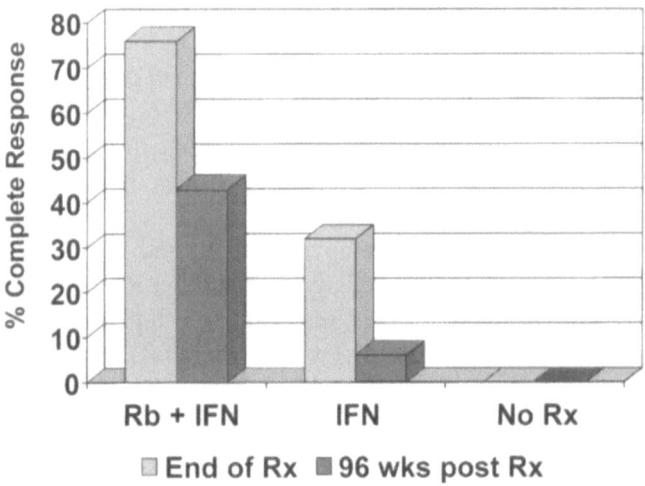

Ribavirin (Rb) + IFNα2a Combination Therapy for Hepatitis C

1200 mg Rb q.d.+ 3 mu IFN t.i.w. *vs.* 3 mu IFN t.i.w. x 24 wks
Complete response = normal ALT and nondetectable HCV RNA
n = 60

□ End of Rx ■ 96 wks post Rx

Fig. 3. Summary of results from a prospective, randomized, controlled clinical trial of ribavirin–interferon combination therapy vs interferon monotherapy, as reported by Lai et al. [70]

in patients with high levels of serum HCV RNA ($>3 \times 10^6$ genome equivalents/ml). The combination offered no advantage over interferon alone in those patients with lower levels of HCV viremia, who overall have a greater chance of a favorable response to interferon monotherapy.

Although the response to interferon–ribavirin combination therapy has not been as impressive in those patients who have previously failed interferon monotherapy, Bellobuono et al. [72] reported both greater end-of-treatment and sustained ALT responses in patients undergoing retreatment with combination therapy, compared with interferon alone. In all studies, the addition of ribavirin to interferon regimens has been relatively well tolerated, with few patients forced to withdraw from therapy due to adverse reactions. However, low-grade hemolysis has been a frequent side effect, and may lead to both anemia and increased intrahepatic iron stores [73]. The latter is a worrisome finding, inasmuch as it could be detrimental to liver function if allowed to reach a significant level.

Although the overall sustained virologic response rates that have been reported with the combination of ribavirin and interferon are still less than satisfactory, the marked benefit that has been noted with the addition of ribavirin to previous interferon therapeutic regimens highlights the potential for combination therapy against this disease. It is particularly noteworthy that the mechanism of action of ribavirin in this setting may not be related to direct suppression of viral replication, but rather to a favorable modulation of the host immune response to the infection. This is suggested by the failure of ribavirin to suppress HCV viremia when administered as monotherapy [66,67], as well as a series of observations concerning the effects of ribavirin on various aspects of the host immune response. It is interesting that the combination of ribavirin and interferon also shows synergy in the treatment of experimental subacute sclerosing panencephalitis (SSPE) virus infections in hamsters [74]. These observations are consistent with a broad effect of ribavirin on the ability of the host immune system to control chronic viral infections.

In animal studies, the course of disease in mice experiencing fulminant hepatitis due to the coronavirus murine hepatitis virus (strain 3) can be attenuated by treatment with ribavirin [75]. This has been shown to be associated with inhibition of macrophage production of TNF and the procoagulant fgl2 prothrombinase. Ribavirin inhibited Th2 cytokine responses, but preserved Th1 cytokine production. Interleukin-6 production has also been shown to modulated by ribavirin in human pulmonary epithelial cells infected with respiratory syncytial virus [76]. The significance of these findings is unclear, however, as is their relationship to the mechanism of action of ribavirin in the setting of combination therapy of hepatitis C. Ribavirin is known to inhibit cellular IMP dehydrogenase [77], and this may influence the ability of cells either to support viral replication or to respond to appropriate immunologic stimuli.

Whatever the mechanism of action of ribavirin when used in combination with interferon for therapy of hepatitis C, the success of this strategy has increased the urgency of the search for additional, specific inhibitors of HCV replication. Although this search is hampered by the absence of tractable cell culture systems that would allow the development of broadbased screens for novel antiviral compounds, significant progress is being made through the use of more sophisticated biochemical screens.

Major Molecular Targets for Antiviral Drug Development—Current Status

NS3 Proteinase

The amino terminal third of the NS3 molecule contains a serine proteinase activity that is active both in *cis* and in *trans* [78,79]. This activity is responsible for the majority of cleavage events occurring within the HCV polyprotein. Thus, inhibition of this activity would have a direct effect on replication of the virus. The complete expression of NS3 proteinase activity is dependent upon the noncovalent assembly of NS3 and NS4a molecules, with the small NS4a component forming an integral part of the proteinase structure. Several pharmaceutical companies have independently solved the crystallographic structure of the proteinase domain of NS3, or the NS3–NS4a proteinase complex [23,80]. Thus, efforts at rational, structure-based drug design are ongoing, along with more conventional screening of compound libraries using biochemical assays of the NS3 proteinase activities. Thus far, however, no highly active inhibitors of this proteinase have yet been described in the literature.

NS3 Helicase

The carboxy terminal two-thirds of the NS3 molecule contains an RNA helicase activity [24,81]. This is almost certainly essential for replication of the viral RNA, although its precise role in the replication cycle is not known. The NS3 helicase domain can be expressed as an active enzyme, permitting the development of in vitro screening assays for compounds with specific inhibitory activities. Like the proteinase domain, the crystallographic structure of the helicase has been solved [25,82]. This will permit the application of structure-based, rational drug design strategies to the refinement of any lead compounds that may be identified in helicase screens.

NS5B RNA Polymerase

The NS5B molecule is the RNA-dependent RNA polymerase that is primarily responsible for the transcription of both the positive and negative strands of viral RNA during virus replication. Several research groups have expressed it in an active form from recombinant cDNA [83,84].

However, activity has been limited to nonspecific, primer-dependent transcription of a variety of RNA transcripts, or to primer-independent terminal transferase activity. No research group has yet reported the reconstruction of an active replicase complex that is capable of specific recognition and initiation of transcription of the 3' end of either the positive- or negative-strand RNA. The reason for this is not clear, although it seems likely that a complex of several viral proteins (and possibly certain cellular proteins as well) might be required for such activity [27]. Thus, while it is possible to screen compound libraries for inhibitors of NS5b primer extension or terminal transferase activities, it is not possible to screen for specific HCV RNA transcription inhibitors. No specific inhibitors have yet been described for the former activities, although there are intense efforts to develop such compounds ongoing within both the pharmaceutical and academic communities.

Internal Ribosome Entry Site

The IRES represents an interesting and completely novel target for antiviral drug development. This segment of the viral genome is essential for the initiation of translation of the polyprotein, and thus inhibition of IRES activity would be expected to have a profound effect on replication of the virus [14]. Recent work suggests that the primary step in the initiation of cap-independent translation of the polyprotein by the IRES is the specific recognition of the 40S ribosome subunit by the IRES [85]. The ability to directly form a binary complex with the 40S subunit in the absence of any canonical or noncanonical translation initiation factor is unique among all eukaryotic RNAs. Similar activities are found only in related IRES segments from other Flaviviridae. This activity should be amenable to inhibition by small molecules which have a high affinity for the RNA structures responsible for this 40S subunit binding activity. A number of pharmaceutical companies are actively pursuing this possibility, but no specific inhibitors of the HCV IRES have yet been described.

Conclusions

Cirrhosis and hepatocellular carcinoma result from longstanding hepatic inflammation related to the persistence of HCV within the liver. Thus, this pathologic process reflects the presence of an active immune response to the infection, yet one which is ineffectual in elimination of the virus. The reasons underlying the ability of this virus to persist in humans despite this immune response are not well understood, but are likely to involve a specific mechanism to "disarm" the immune system. Because of the extreme technical difficulties inherent in HCV vaccine development, present efforts are largely directed at the development of better therapies for chronic hepatitis C. Recent experience with the combination of ribavirin and interferon-α suggest that combination therapies will offer particular advantages in the treatment of this disease. This concept is well supported by earlier experience in the treatment of several other chronic infectious diseases. Thus, the search is on for novel, small molecule inhibitors of HCV replication. This search is complicated by the absence of tractable cell culture systems for propagation of the virus, but a number of biochemical assays have been developed which are now being used as screens for active compounds. It is highly likely that this intense research activity will result in a variety of novel therapeutic agents, and that this will open the door to a new era in the prevention of HCV-related liver disease.

Acknowledgments. This work was supported in part by a grant from the National Institute of Allergy and Infectious Diseases, U19-40035.

References

1. Choo Q-L, Kuo G, Weiner AJ, Overby LR, Bradley DW, Houghton M (1989) Isolation of a cDNA clone derived from a blood-borne non-A, non-B viral hepatitis genome. Science 244:359–362
2. Kuo G, Choo Q-L, Alter HJ, Gitnick GL, Redeker AG, Purcell RH, Miyamura T, Dienstag JL, Alter MJ, Stevens CE, Tegtmeier GE, Bonino F, Colombo M, Lee W-S, Kuo C, Berger K, Shuster JR, Overby LR, Bradley DW, Houghton M (1989) An assay for circulating antibodies to a major etiologic virus of human non-A, non-B hepatitis. Science 244:362–364
3. Alter MJ, Margolis HS, Krawczynski K, Judson FN, Mares A, Alexander WJ, Hu PY, Miller JK, Gerber MA, Sampliner RE, Meeks EL, Beach MJ (1992) The natural history of community-acquired hepatitis C in the United States. N Engl J Med 327:1899–1905
4. Jeffers LJ, Hasan F, de Medina M, Reddy R, Parker T, Silva M, Mendez L, Schiff ER, Manns M, Houghton M, Choo Q-L, Kuo G (1992) Prevalence of antibodies to hepatitis C virus among patients with cryptogenic chronic hepatitis and cirrhosis. Hepatology 15:187–190
5. Saito I, Miyamura T, Ohbayashi A, Harada H, Katayama T, Kikuchi S, Watanabe Y, Koi S, Onji M, Ohta Y, Choo Q-L, Houghton M, Kuo G (1991) Hepatitis C virus

infection is associated with the development of hepatocellular carcinoma. Proc Natl Acad Sci USA 87:6547–6549

6. Lemon SM, Chisari FV, Lai MMC, Mishiro S, Nishioka K, Johnson L (1998) Meeting report: the 19th Joint U.S.-Japan Hepatitis Panel Meeting. In press

7. Alter MJ (1997) Epidemiology of hepatitis C. Hepatology 26 Suppl 1:62S–65S

8. Consensus Development Panel (1997) National Institutes of Health Consensus Development Conference Panel statement: Management of hepatitis C. Hepatology 26 Suppl 1:2S–10S

9. Hsu S-L, Lin Y-F, Chou C-K (1993) Retinoic acid biphasically regulates the gene expression of hepatitis B virus surface antigen in human hepatoma Hep3B cells. J Biol Chem 268:23093–23097

10. Kurosaki M, Enomoto N, Sakamoto N, Tanaka Y, Tang L, Hoshino Y, Izumi Y, Marumo F, Sato C (1995) Detection and analysis of replicating hepatitis C virus RNA in hepatocellular carcinoma tissues. J Hepatol 22:527–535

11. Nishioka K, Mishiro S, Yoshizawa H (1996) Hepatitis C virus infection in the general population of Japan: past and future. Viral Hepatitis Rev 2:199–203

12. Houghton M, Weiner A, Han J, Kuo G, Choo Q-L (1991) Molecular biology of the hepatitis C viruses: implications for diagnosis, development and control of viral disease. Hepatology 14:381–388

13. Major ME, Feinstone SM (1997) The molecular virology of hepatitis C. Hepatology 25:1527–1538

14. Lemon SM, Honda H (1998) Internal ribosome entry sites within the RNA genomes of hepatitis C virus and other flaviviruses. Semin Virol 8:274–288

15. Kolykhalov AA, Feinstone SM, Rice CM (1996) Identification of a highly conserved sequence element at the 3′ terminus of hepatitis C virus genome RNA. J Virol 70:3363–3371

16. Tanaka T, Kato N, Cho M-J, Shimotohno K (1995) A novel sequence found at the 3′ terminus of the hepatitis C virus genome. Biochem Biophys Res Commun 215:744–749

17. Hijikata M, Kato N, Ootsuyama Y, Nakagawa M, Shimotohno K (1991) Gene mapping of the putative structural region of the hepatitis C virus genome by in vitro processing analysis. Proc Natl Acad Sci USA 88:5547–5551

18. Hijikata M, Mizushima H, Akagi T, Mori S, Kakiuchi N, Kato N, Tanaka T, Kimura K, Shimotohno K (1993) Two distinct proteinase activities required for the processing of a putative nonstructural precursor protein of hepatitis C virus. J Virol 67:4665–4675

19. Reed KE, Grakoui A, Rice CM (1995) Hepatitis C virus-encoded NS2–3 protease: Cleavage-site mutagenesis and requirements for bimolecular cleavage. J Virol 69:4127–4136

20. Dubuisson J, Hsu HH, Cheung RC, Greenberg HB, Russell DG, Rice CM (1994) Formation and intracellular localization of hepatitis C virus envelope glycoprotein complexes expressed by recombinant vaccinia and Sindbis viruses. J Virol 68:6147–6160

21. Dubuisson J, Rice CM (1996) Hepatitis C virus glycoprotein folding: disulfide bond formation and association with calnexin. J Virol 70:778–786

22. Failla C, Tomei L, De Francesco R (1994) Both NS3 and NS4A are required for proteolytic processing of hepatitis C virus nonstructural proteins. J Virol 68:3753–3760

23. Kim JL, Morgenstern KA, Lin C, Fox T, Dwyer MD, Landro JA, Chambers SP, Markland W, Lepre CA, O'Malley ET, Harbeson SL, Rice CM, Murcko MA, Caron PR, Thomson JA (1996) Crystal structure of the hepatitis C virus NS3 protease domain complexed with a synthetic NS4A cofactor peptide. Cell 87:343–355

24. Preugschat F, Averett DR, Clarke BE, Porter DJT (1996) A steady-state and pre-steady-state kinetic analysis of the NTPase activity associated with the hepatitis C virus NS3 helicase domain. J Biol Chem 271:24449–24457

25. Yao NH, Hesson T, Cable M, Hong Z, Kwong AD, Le HV, Weber PC (1997) Structure of the hepatitis C virus RNA helicase domain. Nature Struct Biol 4:463–467

26. Asabe SI, Tanji Y, Satoh S, Kaneko T, Kimura K, Shimotohno K (1997) The N-terminal region of hepatitis C virus-encoded NS5A is important for NS4A-dependent phosphorylation. J Virol 71:790–796

27. Ishido S, Fujita T, Hotta H (1998) Complex formation of NS5B with NS3 and NS4A proteins of hepatitis C virus. Biochem Biophys Res Commun 244:35–40

28. Lanford RE, Chavez D, Chisari FV, Sureau C (1995) Lack of detection of negative-strand hepatitis C virus RNA in peripheral blood mononuclear cells and other extrahepatic tissues by the highly strand-specific rTth reverse transcriptase PCR. J Virol 69:8079–8083

29. Anderson DA, Ross BC, Locarnini SA (1988) Restricted replication of hepatitis A virus in cell culture: encapsidation of viral RNA depletes the pool of RNA available for replication. J Virol 62:4201–4206

30. Mizutani T, Kato N, Saito S, Ikeda M, Sugiyama K, Shimotohno S (1996) Characterization of hepatitis C virus replication in cloned cells obtained from a human T-cell leukemia virus type 1-infected cell line, MT-2. J Virol 70:7219–7223

31. Shimizu YK, Iwamoto A, Hijikata M, Purcell RH, Yoshikura H (1992) Evidence for in vitro replication of hepatitis C virus genome in a human T-cell line. Proc Natl Acad Sci USA 89:5477–5481

32. Shimizu YK, Yoshikura H (1994) Multicycle infection of hepatitis C virus in cell culture and inhibition by alpha and beta interferons. J Virol 68:8406–8408

33. Binn LN, Lemon SM, Marchwicki RH, Redfield RR, Gates NL, Bancroft WH (1984) Primary isolation and serial passage of hepatitis A virus strains in primate cell cultures. J Clin Microbiol 20:28–33

34. Bukh J, Miller RH, Purcell RH (1995) Genetic heterogeneity of hepatitis C virus: quasispecies and genotypes. Semin Liv Dis 15:41–63

35. Honda M, Brown EA, Lemon SM (1996) Stability of a stem-loop involving the initiator AUG controls the efficiency of internal initiation of translation on hepatitis C virus RNA. RNA 2:955–968

36. Reynolds JE, Kaminski A, Carroll AR, Clarke BE, Rowlands DJ, Jackson RJ (1996) Internal initiation of translation of hepatitis C virus RNA: the ribosome entry site is at the authentic initiation codon. RNA 2:867–878

37. Rijnbrand RCA, Abbink TEM, Haasnoot PCJ, Spaan WJM, Bredenbeek PJ (1996) The influence of AUG codons in the hepatitis C virus 5' nontranslated region on translation and mapping of the translation initiation window. Virology 226:47–56

38. Kato N, Sekiya H, Ootsuyama Y, Nakazawa T, Hijikata M, Ohkoshi S, Shimotohno K (1993) Humoral immune response to hypervariable region 1 of the putative envelope glycoprotein (gp70) of hepatitis C virus. J Virol 67:3923–3930

39. Shimizu YK, Hijikata M, Iwamoto A, Alter HJ, Purcell RH, Yoshikura H (1994) Neutralizing antibodies against hepatitis C virus and the emergence of neutralization escape mutant viruses. J Virol 68:1494–1500

40. Weiner A, Erickson AL, Kansopon J, Crawford K, Muchmore E, Hughes AL, Houghton M, Walker CM (1995) Persistent hepatitis C virus infection in a chimpanzee is associated with emergence of a cytotoxic T lymphocyte escape variant. Proc Natl Acad Sci USA 92:2755–2759

41. Lesniewski R, Okasinski G, Carrick R, Van Sant C, Desai S, Johnson R, Scheffel J, Moore B, Mushahwar I (1995) Antibody to hepatitis C virus second envelope (HCV-E2) glycoprotein: a new marker of HCV infection closely associated with viremia. J Med Virol 45:415–422

42. Alberti A, Morsica G, Chemello L, Cavalletto D, Noventa F, Pontisso P, Ruol A (1992) Hepatitis C viraemia and liver disease in symptom-free individuals with anti-HCV. Lancet 340:697–698

43. Lesniewski RR, Boardway KM, Casey JM, Desai SM, Devare SG, Leung TK, Mushahwar IK (1993) Hypervariable 5'-terminus of hepatitis C virus E2/NS1 encodes antigenically distinct variants. J Med Virol 40:150–156

44. Matsumoto M, Hsieh TY, Zhu NL, VanArsdale N, Hwang SB, Jeng KS, Gorbalenya AW, Lo SY, Ou JH, Ware CF, Lai MHC (1997) Hepatitis C virus core protein interacts with the cytoplasmic tail of lymphotoxin-receptor. J Virol 71:1301–1309

45. Chen CM, You LR, Hwang LH, Lee YH (1997) Direct interaction of hepatitis C virus core protein with the cellular lymphotoxin-beta receptor modulates the signal pathway of the lymphotoxin-beta receptor. J Virol 71:9417–9426

46. Ray RB, Meyer K, Steele R, Shrivastava A, Aggarwal BB, Ray R (1998) Inhibition of tumor necrosis factor (TNF-alpha)-mediated apoptosis by hepatitis C virus core protein. J Biol Chem 273:2256–2259

47. Ruggieri A, Harada T, Matsuura Y, Miyamura T (1997) Sensitization to Fas-mediated apoptosis by hepatitis C virus core protein. Virology 229:68–76

48. Lerat H, Berby F, Trabaud MA, Vidalin O, Major M, Trepo C, Inchauspe G (1996) Specific detection of hepatitis C virus minus strand RNA in hematopoietic cells. J Clin Invest 97:845–851

49. Enomoto N, Sakuma I, Asahina Y, Kurosaki M, Murakami T, Yamamoto C, Ogura Y, Izumi N, Marumo F, Sato C (1996) Mutations in the nonstructural protein 5A gene and response to interferon in patients with chronic hepatitis C virus 1b infection. N Engl J Med 334:77–81

50. Kurosaki M, Enomoto N, Murakami T, Sakuma I, Asahina Y, Yamamoto C, Ikeda T, Tozuka S, Izumi N, Marumo F, Sato C (1997) Analysis of genotypes and amino acid residues 2209 to 2248 of the NS5A region of hepatitis C virus in relation to the response to interferon-therapy. Hepatology 25:750–753

51. Gale MJ Jr, Korth MJ, Tang NM, Tan SL, Hopkins DA, Dever TE, Polyak SJ, Gretch DR, Katze MG (1997) Evidence that hepatitis C virus resistance to interferon is mediated through repression of the PKR protein kinase by the nonstructural 5A protein. Virology 230:217–227
52. Choo Q-L, Kuo G, Ralston R, Weiner A, Chien D, Van Nest G, Han J, Berger K, Thudium K, Kuo C, Kansopon J, McFarland J, Tabrizi A, Ching K, Moss B, Cummins LB, Houghton M, Muchmore E (1994) Vaccination of chimpanzees against infection by the hepatitis C virus. Proc Natl Acad Sci USA 91:1294–1298
53. Klavinskis LS, Whitton JL, Oldstone MBA (1989) Molecularly engineered vaccine which expresses an immunodominant T-cell epitope induces cytotoxic T lymphocytes that confer protection from lethal virus infection. J Virol 63:4311–4316
54. González A, Esteban JI, Madoz P, Viladomiu L, Genesca J, Muñoz E, Enríquez J, Torras X, Hernández JM, Quer J, Vidal X, Alter HJ, Shih JW, Esteban R, Guardia J (1995) Efficacy of screening donors for antibodies to the hepatitis C virus to prevent transfusion-associated hepatitis: Final report of a prospective trial. Hepatology 22:439–445
55. Nishioka K (1996) Transfusion-transmitted HBV and HCV. Vox Sang 70:4–8
56. Davis GL, Balart LA, Schiff ER, Lindsay K, Bodenheimer HC. Jr, Perillo RP, Carey W, Jacobson IM, Payne J, Dienstag JL, VanThiel DH, Tamburro C, Lefkowitch J, Albrecht J, Meschievitz C, Ortego TJ, Gibas A, Hepatitis Interventional Therapy Group (1989) Treatment of chronic hepatitis C with recombinant interferon alfa: A multicenter randomized, controlled trial. N Engl J Med 321:1501–1506
57. Di Bisceglie AM, Martin P, Kassianides C, Lisker-Melman M, Murray L, Waggoner J, Goodman Z, Banks SM, Hoofnagle JH (1989) Recombinant interferon alfa therapy for chronic hepatitis C: a randomized, double-blind, placebo-controlled trial. N Engl J Med 321:1506–1510
58. Sánchez-Royuela F, Porres JC, Moreno A, Castillo I, Martinez G, Galiana F, Carreño V (1991) High doses of recombinant-interferon or gamma-interferon for chronic hepatitis C: A randomized, controlled trial. Hepatology 13:327–331
59. Nishiguchi S, Kuroki T, Nakatani S, Morimoto H, Takeda T, Nakajima S, Shiomi S, Seki S, Kobayashi K, Otani S (1995) Randomised trial of effects of interferon-α on incidence of hepatocellular carcinoma in chronic active hepatitis C with cirrhosis. Lancet 346:1051–1055
60. Kiyosawa K, Furuta S (1994) Hepatitis C virus and hepatocellular carcinoma. In Reesink HW (Ed) Hepatitis C Virus. Karger, Basel, pp 98–120
61. Mazzella G, Accogli E, Sottili S, Festi D, Orsini M, Salzetta A, Novelli V, Cipolla A, Fabbri C, Pezzoli A, Roda E (1996) Alpha interferon treatment may prevent hepatocellular carcinoma in HCV-related liver cirrhosis. J Hepatol 24:141–147
62. McCormick JB, King IJ, Webb PA, Scribner CL, Craven RB, Johnson KM, Elliott LH, Belmont-Williams R (1986) Lassa fever. Effective therapy with ribavirin. N Engl J Med 314:20–26
63. Smith DW, Frankel LR, Mathers LH, Tang AT, Ariagno RL, Prober CG (1991) A controlled trial of aerosolized ribavirin in infants receiving mechanical ventilation for severe respiratory syncytial virus infection. N Engl J Med 325:24–29

64. Toltzis P, Huang AS (1986) Effect of ribavirin on macromolecular synthesis in vesicular stomatitis virus-infected cells. Antimicrob. Agents Chemother 29:1010–1016

65. Rankin JT Jr, Eppes SB, Antczak JB, Joklik WK (1989) Studies on the mechanism of the antiviral activity of ribavirin against reovirus. Virology 168:147–158

66. Bodenheimer HC Jr, Lindsay KL, Davis GL, Lewis GH, Thung SN, Seeff LB (1997) Tolerance and efficacy of oral ribavirin treatment of chronic hepatitis C: a multicenter trial. Hepatology 26:473–477

67. Di Bisceglie AM, Conjeevaram HS, Fried MW, Sallie R, Park Y, Yurdaydin C, Swain M, Kleiner DE, Mahaney K, Hoofnagle JH, Wright D (1995) Ribavirin as therapy for chronic hepatitis C—a randomized, double-blind, placebo-controlled trial. Ann Intern Med 123:897–903

68. Di Bisceglie AM, Shindo M, Fong T-L, Fried MW, Swain MG, Bergasa NV, Axiotis CA, Waggoner JG, Park Y, Hoofnagle JH (1992) A pilot study of ribavirin therapy for chronic hepatitis C. Hepatology 16:649–654

69. Dusheiko G, Main J, Thomas H, Reichard O, Lee C, Dhillon A, Rassam S, Fryden A, Reesink H, Bassendine M, Norkrans G, Cuypers T, Lelie N, Telfer P, Watson J, Weegink C, Sillikens P, Weiland O (1996) Ribavirin treatment for patients with chronic hepatitis C: results of a placebo-controlled study. J Hepatol 25:591–598

70. Lai MY, Kao JH, Yang PM, Wang JT, Chen PJ, Chan KW, Chu JS, Chen DS (1996) Long-term efficacy of ribavirin plus interferon alfa in the treatment of chronic hepatitis C. Gastroenterology 111:1307–1312

71. Reichard O, Norkrans G, Fryden A, Braconier JH, Sonnerborg A, Weiland O (1998) Randomised, double-blind, placebo-controlled trial of interferon alpha-2b with and without ribavirin for chronic hepatitis C. The Swedish Study Group (see comments). Lancet 351:83–87

72. Bellobuono A, Mondazzi L, Tempini S, Silini E, Vicari F, Ideo G (1997) Ribavirin and interferon-alpha combination therapy vs interferon-alpha alone in the retreatment of chronic hepatitis C: a randomized clinical trial. J Viral Hepatal 4:185–191

73. Di Bisceglie AM, Bacon BR, Kleiner DE, Hoofnagle JH (1994) Increase in hepatic iron stores following prolonged therapy with ribavirin in patients with chronic hepatitis C. J Hepatol 21:1109–1112

74. Takahashi T, Hosoya M, Kimura K, Ohno K, Mori S, Takahashi K, Shigeta S (1998) The cooperative effect of interferon-alpha and ribavirin on subacute sclerosing panencephalitis (SSPE) virus infections, in vitro and in vivo (In Process Citation). Antiviral Res 37:29–35

75. Ning Q, Brown D, Parodo J, Cattral M, Gorczynski R, Cole E, Fung L, Ding JW, Liu MF, Rotstein O, Phillips MJ, Levy G (1998) Ribavirin inhibits viral-induced macrophage production of TNF, IL-1, the procoagulant fgl2 prothrombinase and preserves Th1 cytokine production but inhibits Th2 cytokine response [In Process Citation]. J Immunol 160:3487–3493

76. Jiang Z, Kunimoto M, Patel JA (1998) Autocrine regulation and experimental modulation of interleukin-6 expression by human pulmonary epithelial cells infected with respiratory syncytial virus (In Process Citation). J Virol 72:2496–2499

77. Yamada Y, Natsumeda Y, Weber G (1988) Action of the active metabolites of tiazofurin and ribavirin on purified IMP dehydrogenase. Biochemistry 27:2193–2196
78. Grakoui A, McCourt DW, Wychowski C, Feinstone SM, Rice CM (1993) Characterization of the hepatitis C virus-encoded serine proteinase: Determination of proteinase-dependent polyprotein cleavage sites. J Virol 67:2832–2843
79. Tanji Y, Hijikata M, Hirowatari Y, Shimotohno K (1994) Hepatitis C virus polyprotein processing: kinetics and mutagenic analysis of serine proteinase-dependent cleavage. J Virol 68:8418–8422
80. Love RA, Parge HE, Wickersham JA, Hostomsky Z, Habuka N, Moomraw EW, Adachi T, Hostomska Z (1996) The crystal structure of hepatitis C virus NS3 proteinase reveals a trypsin-like fold and a structural zinc binding site. Cell 87:331–342
81. Tai CL, Chi WK, Chen DS, Hwang LH (1996) The helicase activity associated with hepatitis C virus nonstructural protein 3 (NS3). J Virol 70:8477–8484
82. Kim JL, Morgenstern KA, Griffith JP, Dwyer MD, Thomson JA, Murcko MA, Lin C, Caron PR (1998) Hepatitis C virus NS3 RNA helicase domain with a bound oligonucleotide: the crystal structure provides insights into the mode of unwinding. Structure 6:89–100
83. Behrens SE, Tomei L, De Francesco R (1996) Identification and properties of the RNA-dependent RNA polymerase of hepatitis C virus. EMBO J 15:12–22
84. Lohmann V, Korner F, Herian U, Bartenschlager R (1997) Biochemical properties of hepatitis C virus NS5B RNA-dependent RNA polymerase and identification of amino acid sequence motifs essential for enzymatic activity. J Virol 71:8416–8428
85. Pestova TV, Shatsky IN, Fletcher SP, Jackson RJ, Hellen CU (1998) A prokaryotic-like mode of cytoplasmic eukaryotic ribosome binding to the initiation codon during internal translation initiation of hepatitis C and classical swine fever virus RNAs. Genes Dev 12:67–83

Different Quasispecies of Hepatitis C Virus in Human Serum, Peripheral Blood Mononuclear Cells, and Liver

Keisuke Hino, Michiari Okuda, Masaaki Korenaga, Yuhki Yamaguchi, Yoshiharu Katoh, and Kiwamu Okita

Introduction

Several lines of evidence suggest that hepatitis C virus (HCV) can infect peripheral blood mononuclear cells (PBMCs) in persistently infected individuals on the basis of specific detection of negative-strand hepatitis C virus (HCV) RNA in PBMCs by reverse transcription–polymerase chain reaction (RT-PCR) and in situ hybridization [1–5]. However, direct information on the pathogenic implication of HCV infection of PBMCs is limited.

HCV comprises a heterogeneous mixture of genetically different but closely related variants known as "quasispecies" [6]. The most heterogeneous domains of the HCV genome are present within the putative envelope 2 (E2) region and are referred to as hypervariable regions (HVR 1 and HVR 2) [7,8]. Although this quasispecies nature of HCV is generated by the limited fidelity of RNA replication, host immunity, especially the humoral immune response, is thought to be one of the important driving forces in the sequence variations of the HVR of HCV [9–11]. We therefore compared the complexity of HVR 1 quasispecies of the HCV genome in serum, PBMCs, and liver, to assess the pathogenic implication of HCV infection in PBMCs.

Patients and Methods

Eight Japanese patients with type C chronic liver disease (5 men and 3 women, aged 27–58 years, with a mean age of 44) who had HCV type 1b RNA were included in this study (Table 1). None received any antiviral

First Department of Internal Medicine, Yamaguchi University, School of Medicine, 1144 Kogushi, Ube, Yamaguchi 755, Japan

Table 1. Clinical characteristics of patients

| Patient | Age | Sex | ALT | Histology[a] | | Genotype | HCV RNA Level (log Eq/ml)[b] |
				Grading	Staging		
1	58	M	173	Severe	3	1b	6.5
2	47	F	50	Minimal	1	1b	7.0
3	51	F	73	Severe	4	1b	6.4
4	27	M	50	Minimal	1	1b	7.0
5	34	F	21	Minimal	1	1b	5.8
6	45	M	35	Mild	1	1b	<5.5
7	35	M	83	Moderate	2	1b	6.2
8	45	M	151	Minimal	1	1b	6.6

ALT, alanine aminotransferase; HCV, hepatitis C virus.
[a] Histologic diagnoses were made according to recently devised criteria for grading inflammatory activity (minimal, mild, moderate, and severe) and for staging fibrosis (F1, F2, F3, and F4).
[b] HCV RNA level was measured by branched DNA probe assay.

therapy prior to the study. Liver biopsy was performed on all patients for diagnostic purposes.

Serum and PBMC samples were obtained on the same day as liver biopsy. Biopsy specimens were divided into two portions: one was for light microscopy and the other was used for detection of HCV RNA. The PBMCs were separated from 10 ml of heparinized blood by density gradient centrifugation with Leuco PREP, washed three times with RPMI 1640 culture medium, and stored at −80°C until use, as were serum and liver specimens.

Genotyping of HCV RNA

HCV genotypes were determined by a modification of the method of Okamoto et al. [12].

Measurement of HCV RNA in Serum

The HCV RNA level in all serum samples was measured by signal amplification with a branched DNA probe assay.

Cross-mixing Test and Treatment of PBMCs with Trypsin-EDTA and RNase A

To eliminate false positives in PBMCs samples due to contamination by serum HCV RNA, the following experiments were carried out. PBMCs obtained from five healthy controls were incubated with serum including a high titer of HCV RNA at room temperature for 30 min. After centrifugation, PBMCs were treated with trypsin and EDTA, and incubated at 37°C for 20 min. Subsequently, 50 µl of RNase A was added and the cell suspension was incubated at 37°C for 15 min. Thus, PBMCs from healthy controls that had been preincubated with HCV RNA-positive serum were subjected to RT-PCR with or without treatment by trypsin-EDTA and RNase A. PBMCs from patients were also treated with trypsin-EDTA and RNase A, then the HVR 1 was amplified by RT-PCR as described below.

Detection of Negative-strand HCV RNA

Negative strands were detected by synthesis of cDNA with the outer sense primer deduced from the 5′-noncoding region. RNA extracted from serum and PBMCs was heated at 70°C for 5 min and subsequently kept on ice. cDNA was synthesized using the same parameters and conditions as for detection of the positive strand, followed by heating in boiling water for 60 min for inactivation of reverse transcriptase. Subsequently, all samples were treated with RNase A to digest total RNA for prevention of possible reverse transcription and subsequent amplification of positive-strand HCV RNA by Taq polymerase.

Amplification of HVR 1 by RT-PCR

RNA extracted from serum, PBMCs (10^6–10^7 cells), or homogenized liver tissue was reverse transcribed, and DNA fragments containing the HVR 1 were amplified, as described previously [13].

Cloning and Sequencing

The PCR products were subcloned into pGEM-T vector, as described previously [14]. Insertions of DNA fragments were confirmed by PCR, using universal primers. After purification of these PCR products, 8 to 11 subclones per specimen (serum, PBMCs, or liver tissue) were sequenced in both directions with an ABI 373S sequencer.

Results

PBMCs from healthy controls were all negative for HCV RNA after incubation with HCV RNA-positive serum and treatment with trypsin-EDTA and RNase A treatment, but those from one healthy control were positive for HCV RNA without treatment. In contrast, PBMCs from all patients were positive for HCV RNA irrespective of treatment with trypsin-EDTA and RNase A. Negative-strand HCV RNA was detected in PBMCs in 6 patients (patients 1–4, 7, and 8) but was not detected in serum in any patient.

Differences in the complexity of HVR 1 quasispecies were found between serum, PBMCs, and liver in all patients, and the predominant clones from each source were mutually different in patient 8 (Fig. 1). The percentage difference in amino acid sequences between the predominant clone and another minor clone ranged from 3.7% to 59.3% (Fig. 1). Amino acid sequences common to serum and PBMCs were found in 4 patients (patients 2, 3, 7, and 8); those common to serum and liver in 3 patients (patients 1, 3, and 4); and those common to PBMCs and liver in 3 patients (patients 2, 4, and 5). Amino acid sequences unique to serum existed in all patients; those unique to PBMCs, or liver in 6 patients (patients 1, 3, 4, 5, 7, and 8) and in 7 patients (patients 1–4, 6, 7, and 8), respectively. The complexity of HVR 1 quasispecies, defined as the number of distinct amino acid sequences, was 5.4 ± 1.8 in serum ($P = 0.0082$, vs PBMCs), 2.9 ± 1.0 in PBMCs, and 3.4 ± 1.0 in liver.

Discussion

A cross-mixing test of PBMCs from healthy controls with HCV RNA-positive serum showed false detection of HCV RNA in PBMCs due to the adsorption of HCV from serum in a control, and also demonstrated that this contamination could be eliminated by treatment with trypsin-EDTA and subsequently with RNase A. In addition, negative-strand HCV RNA was found in PBMCs, but not in serum. These findings suggested that HCV replication might take place in PBMCs.

Our study demonstrated differences in the complexity and specific sequences of HVR 1 quasispecies among serum, PBMCs, and liver, which

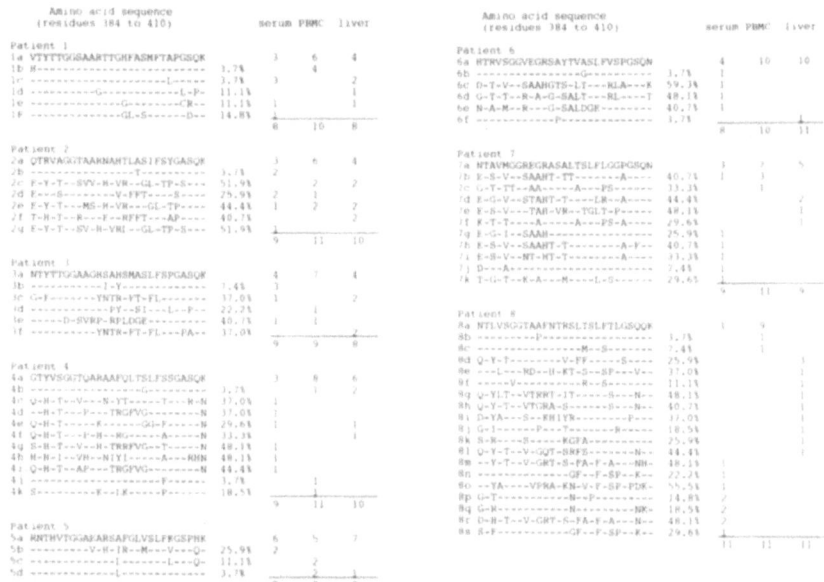

Fig. 1. Hypervariable region (HVR) 1 amino acid sequence of hepatitis C virus (HCV) and numbers of clones obtained from serum, peripheral blood mononuclear cells (*PBMCs*), and liver in all patients. Eight to 11 subclones were obtained from each tissue. Identical clones are represented by combination of a number and a letter such as *1a*, *1b*, or *1c*. The percent amino acid difference of each clone was calculated on the basis of the amino acid sequence of the predominant clone (amino acid sequence in the uppermost line). Amino acid residues are represented by a single-letter code and numbered according to the sequence of HCV-J4 [15]. Horizontal bars indicate amino acids identical to those of the predominant clone

is also indicative of infection of PBMCs by HCV. These findings are compatible with the observations that different quasispecies of HVR 1 existed in serum, PBMCs, and liver in chimpanzees that had been inoculated with HCV strain H77 [16] and in patients with chronic hepatitis C [17]. As HVR 1 is the most heterogeneous domain in the HCV genome, the possibility should be taken into consideration that artificial quasispecies may be generated during RT-PCR [18]. We previously demonstrated high homology as well as considerable differences in HVR 1 quasispecies between immune and nonimmune complexes, using exactly the same methods as in the present study [14]. In addition, another five subclones from each tissue were examined for the HVR 1 quasispecies in patient 8, who showed the most heterogeneous quasispecies, but the results were almost the same. These results indicated that the different complexity of HVR 1 quasispecies found in each tissue in all patient was unlikely to be the result of artificial substitution of the virus sequence.

The heterogeneity of HVR 1 quasispecies observed in one patient (12.5%), who also showed differences in the predominant clone in each tissue, might result in or result from different neutralization with antibodies to HVR 1, because antibodies to HVR 1 have been shown to have neutralizing activity and are found in persistently infected patients [9,19,20]. Although such an event does not appear to occur so frequently, it is possible that neutralization escape mutants, which have already disappeared from the liver, persist in PBMCs. The tendency of the complexity of HVR 1 quasispecies to be greater in serum than in PBMCs or liver, and the presence of HCV variants common to serum and PBMCs, suggests that the quasispecies of circulating HCV are derived from HCV in both PBMCs and liver. This also implies the potential release of virions from PBMCs, even though there is no evidence as yet of the active release of virions from PBMCs. On the other hand, it was uncertain why certain variants were present in serum, but not in PBMCs or liver, in all patients. These results were consistent with those of Maggi et al. [17] in that variants unique to serum were found in 7 of 10 patients. This does not necessarily imply that serum-specific sequences are derived from yet another site, i.e., not liver or PBMCs. This could occur if such variants represent a very small proportion of the quasispecies in PBMCs or liver, but are actively released.

References

1. Wang JT, Sheu JC, Lin JT, Wang TH, Chen DS (1992) Detection of replicative form hepatitis C virus RNA in peripheral blood mononuclear cells. J Infect Dis 166:1167–1169
2. Willems M, Peerlinck K, Moshage H, Deleu I, Van den Eynde C, Vermylen J, Yap SH (1994) Hepatitis C virus-RNAs in plasma and in peripheral blood mononuclear cells of hemophiliacs with chronic hepatitis C: evidence for viral replication in peripheral blood mononuclear cells. J Med Virol 42:272–278
3. Muller HM, Pfaff E, Goeser T, Kallinwski B, Solbach C, Thielman L (1993) Peripheral blood leukocytes serve as a possible extrahepatic site for hepatitis C virus replication. J Gen Virol 74:669–676
4. Moldvay BJ, Deny P, Pol S, Brechot C, Lamas E (1994) Detection of hepatitis C virus RNA in peripheral blood mononuclear cells of infected patients by in situ hybridization. Blood 83:269–273

5. Lerat H, Berby F, Trabaud MA, Vidalin O, Major M, Trepo C, Inchauspe G (1996) Specific detection of hepatitis C virus strand RNA in hematopoietic cells. J Clin Invest 97:845-851

6. Martell M, Esteban J, Ouer J, Genesca J, Weiner A, Esteban R, Guardia J, et al (1992) Hepatitis C virus (HCV) circulates as a population of different but closely related genomes: quasispecies nature of HCV genome distribution. J Virol 66:3225-3229

7. Hijikata M, Kato N, Ootsuyama Y, Nakagawa M, Ohkoshi S, Shimotohno K (1991) Hypervariable region in the putative glycoprotein of hepatitis C virus. Biochem Biophys Res Commun 175:220-228

8. Kato N, Ootsuyama Y, Ohkoshi S, Nakazawa T, Sekiya H, Hijikata M, Shimotohno K (1992) Characterization of hypervariable regions in the putative envelope protein of hepatitis C virus. Biochem Biophys Res Commun 189:119-127

9. Kato N, Ootsuyama Y, Sekiya H, Ohkoshi S, Nakazawa T, Hijikata M, Shimotohno K (1994) Genetic drift in hypervariable region 1 of the viral genome in persistent hepatitis C virus infection. J Virol 68:4776-4784

10. Kurosaki M, Enomoto N, Marumo F, Sato C (1993) Rapid sequence variation of the hypervariable region of hepatitis C virus during the course of chronic infection. Hepatology 18:1293-1299

11. Lawal Z, Petric J, Wong VS, Alexander GJA, Allain JP (1997) Hepatitis C virus genomic variability in untreated and immunosuppressed patients. Virology 228:107-111

12. Okamoto H, Sugiyama Y, Okada S, Kurai K, Akahane Y, Sugai Y, Tanaka T, et al (1992) Typing hepatitis C virus by polymerase chain with type-specific primers: application to clinical surveys and tracing infectious sources. J Gen Virol 73: 673-679

13. Fujii K, Hino K, Okazaki M, Okuda M, Kondoh S, Okita K (1996) Differences in hypervariable region 1 quasispecies of hepatitis C virus between human serum and peripheral blood mononuclear cells. Biochem Biophys Res Commun 225:771-776

14. Korenaga M, Hino K, Okazaki M, Okuda M, Okita K (1997) Differences in hypervariable region 1 quasispecies between immune complexed and non-immune complexed hepatitis C virus particles. Biochem Biophys Res Commun 240:677-682

15. Okamoto H, Kojima M, Okada S, Yoshizawa H, Iizuka H, Tanaka T, Muchmore EE, et al (1992) Genetic drift of hepatitis C virus during an 8.2-year infection in a chimpanzee: variability and stability. Virology 190:894-899

16. Shimizu YK, Igarashi H, Kanematsu T, Fujiwara K, Wong DC, Purcell RH, Yoshikura H (1997) Sequence analysis of the hepatitis C virus genome recovered from serum, liver, and peripheral blood mononuclear cells of infected chimpanzees. J Virol 71:5769-5773

17. Maggi F, Fornai C, Linda M, Giorgi M, Morrica A, Pistello M, Cammarota G, et al (1997) Differences in hepatitis C virus quasispecies composition between liver, peripheral blood mononuclear cells and plasma. J Gen Virol 78:1521-1525

18. Smith DB, McAllister J, Casino C, Simmonds P (1997) Virus "quasispecies": making a mountain out of a molehill? J Gen Virol 78:1511-1519

19. Shimizu YK, Hijikata M, Iwamoto A, Alter HJ, Purcell RH, Yoshikura H (1994) Neutralizing antibodies against hepatitis C virus and the emergence of neutralization escape mutant viruses. J Virol 68:1494–1500

20. Farci P, Alter HJ, Wong DC, Miller RH, Govindarajan S, Engle R, Shapiro M, et al (1994) Prevention of hepatitis C virus infection in chimpanzees after antibody-mediated in vitro neutralization. Proc Natl Acad Sci USA 91:7792–7796

High Prevalence of HCV Infection in Patients with Oral Cancer and Oral Precancerous Lesion

MICHIO SATA[1], YUMIKO NAGAO[2], TADAMITSU KAMEYAMA[2], and KYUICHI TANIKAWA[1]

Introduction

Hepatitis C virus (HCV) leads to serious consequences such as liver cirrhosis and hepatocellular carcinoma. Other than liver disease, HCV infection is associated with various extrahepatic manifestations and immunological disorders which include membranoproliferative glomerulonephritis, cryoglobulinemia, autoimmune thyroiditis, Sjögren syndrome, malignant lymphoma, and lichen planus [1–3]. Many authors have reported a relationship between pathogenesis of lichen planus and HCV infection [4–6]. We reported evidence of the high prevalence of HCV infection in patients with oral cancer or oral lichen planus (OLP) [7–18].

OLP, which is associated with oral malignancy, is an inflammatory and intractable disease with a long course associated with chronic hyperkeratosis. OLP affects skin and mucosa of squamous cell origin. The prevalence of OLP varies from 0.7% to 2.2% in the general population. The disease seems to be predominantly present in women and in those of middle age or older. The most common and typical pattern is one of well-defined white striae affecting the buccal mucosa symmetrically. Erosive or bullous types of OLP generally cause intensive contact pains. The histopathologic appearance of the main characteristics is a band-like lymphocytic infiltrate directly adjacent to and invading into the epithelium.

[1] Second Department of Medicine and [2] Department of Oral Surgery, Kurume University School of Medicine, 67 Asahi-machi, Kurume, Fukuoka 830-0011, Japan

Subjects and Methods

We analyzed the relationship between oral cancer, precancerous lesions, and HCV infection [7,8,15–17].

Our first subject group consisted of 100 oral cancer and 45 OLP patients (Group 1). The oral cancer patients had been admitted to the Department of Oral Surgery of the Kurume University School of Medicine from January 1989 to October 1993 for the surgical resection of newly diagnosed oral cancer; the OLP patients visited the Department of Oral Surgery from November 1993 to April 1994. Serum hepatitis B virus surface antigen (HBsAg) was assayed by an enzyme immunoassay (EIA) using Quik Test (Mizuho Medy, Tosu, Japan) according to the manufacturer's instructions. Antibodies to HCV (anti-HCV) were assayed with the second generation of anti-HCV assay passive hemagglutination (PHA) kit (Dainabbott, Tokyo, Japan) according to the manufacturer's instructions. HCV RNA in sera was determined by HCV-specific oligonucleotides and reverse transcription–nested polymerase chain reaction (RT-nested PCR).

We next investigated the prevalence of HCV infection in patients with head and neck squamous cell carcinoma (SCC) in Japan. This study design was based on a prospective cohort at the national level. The subject group included sera from 305 patients with head and neck SCC and 276 patients with nonmalignant disease (the control group) from five geographically distinct institutions (Group 2). The five institutions involved in this study were the Hokkaido University School of Dentistry at Sapporo, the Nihon University School of Dentistry, Kanagawa Cancer Center, the Kurume University School of Medicine, and the Kumamoto University School of Medicine. All sera were examined for antibodies to HCV (anti-HCV) and serum HCV RNA.

The incidence of oral precancerous lesions among the inhabitants in an HCV hyperendemic area were investigated. Two oral surgeons examined the oral lesions of 685 adult inhabitants in H town [19], a hyperendemic area of HCV infection (Group 3). All sera were examined for antibodies to HCV (anti-HCV) and serum HCV RNA.

Finally, we investigated the existence of HCV RNA in 17 oral cancer tissues and 19 OLP tissues from subjects with and without antibody to HCV (Group 4).

Results and Discussion

Incidence of HCV Infection in Patients with OLP and Oral Cancer in Kurume University Hospital

Anti-HCV was detected in sera from 24 of the 100 (24%) patients with oral cancer, in 28 of 45 (62%) OLP patients, and in 11 of 104 (10.6%) control patients (Fig. 1). Disease of the control group was nonmalignant disease while receiving dental treatment at the Department of Oral Surgery. All of the oral cancer patients were HBsAg-negative; on the other hand, HBsAg was positive in only 4 of 45 OLP patients (8.9%).

Liver disease was observed in 35 (78%) of 45 OLP patients, including chronic hepatitis C (22 cases, 49%), chronic hepatitis B and C (1), chronic hepatitis B (3), HCV-related liver cirrhosis (2), HCV-related hepatocellular carcinoma (2), alcoholic liver disease (3), and constitutional jaundice (1) (Table 1). One patient was an asymptomatic HCV carrier. Both anti-HCV and HCV RNA were detected in the majority of patients with HCV-related liver disease. The remaining 10 (22%) patients were free from liver

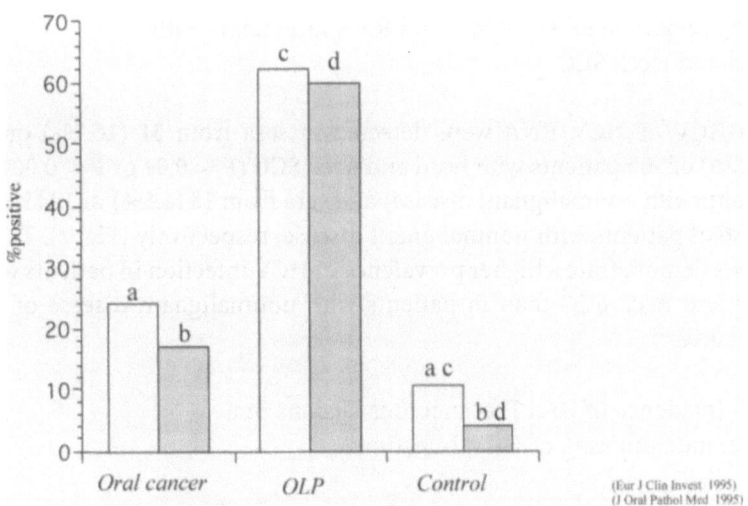

Fig. 1. Prevalence of hepatitis C virus (HCV) infection in oral cancer and oral lichen planus (*OLP*). *Open bars*, anti-HCV; *stippled bars*, HCV RNA. *a*, $P < 0.05$; *b*, $P < 0.05$; *c*, $P < 0.00001$; *d*, $P < 0.0000001$

Table 1. Liver disease of 45 patients with oral lichen planus (OLP)

Diagnosis	No. of patients (%)
Liver disease	35 (77.8)
Chronic hepatitis C	22 (48.9)
Chronic hepatitis B and C	1 (2.2)
HCV-related liver cirrhosis	2 (4.4)
HCV-related hepatocellular carcinoma	2 (4.4)
Chronic hepatitis B	3 (6.7)
Asymptomatic HCV carrier	1 (2.2)
Alcoholic liver disease	3 (6.7)
alcoholic liver disease	1
liver cirrhosis	1
fatty liver	1
Constitutional jaundice	1 (2.2)
No evidence of liver disease	10 (22.2)

disease, and negative for HBsAg, anti-HCV and HCV RNA. However, our results showed that OLP was observed not only in patients with severe liver dysfunction but also in patients without it.

High Prevalence of Anti-HCV and RNA in Patients with Head and Neck SCC

Anti-HCV or HCV RNA were detected in sera from 51 (16.7%) or 35 (11.5%) of 305 patients with head and neck SCC ($P < 0.01$ or $P < 0.001$ vs patients with nonmalignant disease) and sera from 18 (6.5%) or 10 (3.6%) of 276 of patients with nonmalignant disease, respectively (Fig. 2). These results demonstrate a higher prevalence of HCV infection in patients with head and neck SCC than in patients with nonmalignant disease of the same area.

High Incidence of Oral Precancerous Lesions in a Hyperendemic Area of HCV Infection

To clarify the rate of oral cancer and precancerous lesions in patients with HCV infection, we analyzed the relationship between these diseases and HCV infection, involving the mass screening of inhabitants of a specific geographic area. A total of 685 adult inhabitants in H town, a hyperendemic area of HCV infection, participated in the study.

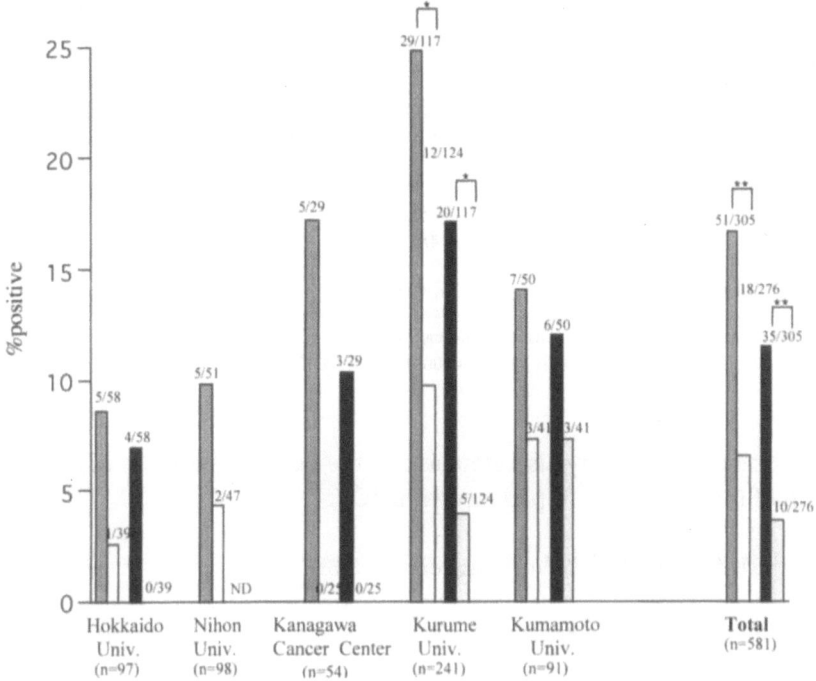

Fig. 2. Head and neck squamous cell carcinoma (SCC) and HCV infection in Japan: prospective cohort at the national level. Prevalence of serum anti-HCV and HCV RNA in 305 patients with head and neck SCC and 276 patients with non-malignant disease (control). The chi-square test was used for statistical analyses. *Dark-gray bars*, anti-HCV in SCC; *white bars*, anti-HCV in control; *black bars*, HCV RNA in SCC; *light-gray bars*, HCV RNA in control. $*P < 0.01$; $**P < 0.001$

OLP, leukoedema, or leukoplakia were observed in 10 (1.5%), 82 (12%), or 47 (6.9%) subjects, respectively (Table 2). The incidences of OLP, leukoedema, and leukoplakia in the subjects with HCV infection were significantly higher than in those without HCV. Although no one had oral cancer, these results indicated that HCV may play an important role in oral cancer and related precancerous lesions.

While there is no doubt that a small percentage of leukoplakia cases are premalignant and some may be invasive carcinoma at presentation, leukoedema is an abnormality of the buccal mucosa which clinically resembles early leukoplakia, but appears to differ from it in certain respects.

Table 2. Subject characteristics of oral precancerous lesions in a hyperendemic area of hepatitis C virus (HCV) infection

Clinical features	Total	OLP	Leukoedema	Leukoplakia
Subjects (%)	685	10 (1.5)	82 (12.0)	47 (6.9)
Age (years) (mean ± SD)	56.1 ± 16.1	60.8 ± 11.6	62.0 ± 15.7	58.1 ± 16.5
Sex (male/female)	295/390	8/2	58/24	31/16
Anti-HCV (+) (%)	84 (12.3)	4/84 (4.8)	18/84 (21.4)	18/84 (21.4)
HCV RNA (+) (%)	61 (8.9)	4/61 (6.6) [a]	14/61 (23.0) [a]	15/61 (24.6) [d]
Anti-HCV (−) and HCV RNA (−) (%)	591 (86.3)	6/591 (1.0) [b]	60/591 (10.2) [c]	26/591 (4.4) [e]

SD, standard deviation; (+), positive; (−), negative.

[a] $P < 0.01$; [b] $P < 0.001$; [c] $P < 0.01$; [d] $P < 0.000001$; [e] $P < 0.0000001$, chi-squared test.

Moreover, our study also emphasized the need for periodic examination of the oral cavity in patients with HCV.

HCV RNA Detection in Oral Cancer and OLP Tissue

We investigated the existence of HCV RNA in 17 oral cancer and 19 OLP tissues from subjects with and without antibody to HCV (Table 3). A sensitive RT-nested PCR detected HCV RNA in all tissues from antibody-positive patients. In oral cancer tissues, positive and negative HCV RNA strands were observed in 7 (7/7, 100%) and 5 (5/7, 71.4%) tissues, respectively. Neither positive nor negative strands were present in oral cancer and nonmalignant tissue from those who were HCV antibody-negative.

In OLP tissues, a sensitive RT-PCR detected HCV RNA in 13 of 14 tissues from antibody-positive patients. Positive and negative HCV RNA strands were observed in 13 (92.9%) and 3 (21.4%) OLP tissues, respectively. On the other hand, neither positive nor negative strands were present in OLP tissue from those who were HCV antibody-negative. These results indicate that HCV persists and replicates in oral cancer and OLP lesions, suggesting a pathological role of HCV in these diseases.

Immunohistological Staining in OLP Tissues

The expression of HCV envelope protein was determined by immuno-histochemistory using a monoclonal antibody to HCV envelope protein. Envelope antigen was expressed on the cytoplasm of mucoepidermis cells.

Table 3. Clinical information and incidence of HCV infection for 17 oral cancer and 19 OLP patients

Diagnosis	No. of patients	HCV RNA in serum	HCV RNA in tissue (+) stand/(−) strand	No. of patients
Oral cancer				
Anti-HCV-positive	7	+	+/+	5
		+	+/−	2
Anti-HCV-negative	10	−	−/−	10
Nonmalignant disease				
Anti-HCV-negative	4	−	−/−	4
OLP				
Liver disease				
HCV infectious disease				
HCV carrier	1	+	+/+	1
Chronic hepatitis C	10	+	+/−	6
		+	−/−	1
		+	+/−	1
		+	+/+	2
HCV-Related liver cirrhosis	3	+	+/−	2
		−	+/−	1
Non-HCV infectious disease				
Chronic hepatitis B	1	−	−/−	1
Alcoholic liver cirrhosis	1	−	−/−	1
Fatty liver	1	−	−/−	1
No evidence of liver disease	2	−	−/−	2

+, HCV RNA-positive; −, HCV RNA-negative.

Conclusion

(1) We have reported extrahepatic manifestations which include OLP and oral cancer. We found new evidence for the high prevalence of antibody and RNA of HCV in oral cancer and OLP patients in the Northern Kyusyu district of Japan, where the prevalence of anti-HCV is the highest in the country. The results in this study would call attention to physicians and dentists to investigate liver disease and HCV infection in patients with oral cancer and OLP.

(2) We have investigated a prevalence of HCV infection in patients with head and neck SCC in Japan. The results demonstrate, at the national level, a higher prevalence of HCV infection in patients with head and neck SCC than in patients with nonmalignant disease of the same area.

(3) We have investigated the incidence of oral precancerous lesions among the inhabitants in an HCV hyperendemic area. The incidences of OLP, leukoedema, and leukoplakia in subjects with HCV infection were significantly higher than in those without HCV. These results indicate that HCV persists and replicates in oral cancer and OLP lesions, suggesting a pathological role of HCV in these diseases, although the mechanisms are unclear.

(4) Taken together, our results indicated that HCV may play an important role in oral cancer and related precancerous lesions. Moreover, our study also emphasized the need for periodic examination of the oral cavity in patients with HCV.

References

1. Johnson RJ, Gretch DR, Yamabe H, et al (1993) Membranoproliferative glomerulonephritis associated with hepatitis C virus infection. N Engl J Med 328:465–470
2. Gumber SC, Chopra S (1995) Hepatitis C: a multifaced disease. Ann Intern Med 123:615–620
3. Ferric C, Civita LL, Monti M, et al (1995) Can type C hepatitis infection be complicated by malignant lymphoma? Lancet 346:1426–1427
4. Jubert C, Pawlotsky JM, Pouget F, et al (1994) Lichen planus and hepatitis C virus-related chronic active hepatitis. Arch Dermatol 130:73–76
5. Gandolfo S, Carbone M, Carrozzo M, Gallo V (1994) Oral lichen planus and hepatitis C virus (HCV) infection: is there a relationship? A report of 10 cases. J Oral Pathol Med 23:119–122

6. Carrozzo M, Gandolfo S, Carbone M, et al (1996) Hepatitis C virus infection in Italian patients with oral lichen planus: a prospective case-control study. J Oral Pathol Med 25:527–533

7. Nagao Y, Sata M, Tanikawa K, Itoh K, Kameyama T (1995) High prevalence of hepatitis C virus antibody and RNA in patients with oral cancer. J Oral Pathol Med 24:354–360

8. Nagao Y, Sata M, Tanikawa K, Itoh K, Kameyama T (1995) Lichen planus and hepatitis C virus in the Northern Kyushu region of Japan. Eur J Clin Invest 25:910–914

9. Nagao Y, Sata M, Tanikawa K, Kameyama T (1995) A case of oral lichen planus with chronic hepatitis C successfully treated by glycyrrhizin. J J A Infect Dis 69:940–943

10. Nagao Y, Sata M, Fukuizumi K, Harada H, Kameyama T (1996) Oral cancer and hepatitis C virus (HCV): can HCV alone cause oral cancer? A case report. Kurume Med J 43:97–100

11. Nagao Y, Sata M, Itoh K, Tanikawa K, Kameyama T (1996) Quantitative analysis of HCV RNA and genotype in patients with chronic hepatitis C accompanied by oral lichen planus. Eur J Clin Invest 26:495–498

12. Nagao Y, Sata M, Suzuki H, Tanikawa K, Itoh K, Kameyama T (1996) Effectiveness of glycyrrhizin for oral lichen planus in patients with chronic HCV infection. J Gastroenterol 31:691–695

13. Nagao Y, Sata M, Ide T, et al (1996) Development and exacerbation of oral lichen planus during and after interferon therapy for hepatitis C. Eur J Clin Invest 26:1171–1174

14. Nagao Y, Sata M, Tanikawa K, Kameyama T (1997) Immunological evaluation in oral lichen planus with chronic hepatitis C. J Gastroenterol 32:324–329

15. Nagao Y, Sata M, Itoh K, et al (1997) High prevalence of hepatitis C virus antibody and RNA in patients with head and neck squamous cell carcinoma. Hepatol Res 7:206–211

16. Nagao Y, Sata M, Fukuizumi K, Tanikawa K, Kameyama T (1997) High incidence of oral precancerous lesions in a hyperendemic area of hepatitis C virus infection. Hepatol Res 8:173–177

17. Nagao Y, Sata M, Kameyama T (1998) Hepatitis C virus RNA detection in oral lichen planus tissue. Am J Gastroenterol 93:850

18. Yoshida M, Nagao Y, Sata M, Kusukawa J, Kameyma T (1998) Multiple primary neoplasms and HCV infection in oral cancer patients. Hepatol Res: in press

19. Yamakawa Y, Sata M, Suzuki H, Noguchi S, Tanikawa K (1996) Higher elimination rate of hepatitis C virus among women. J Viral Hepatitis 3:317–321

Hepatitis C Virus Nonstructural Region 5A Protein: A Potent Transcriptional Activator

Naoya Kato, Keng-Hsin Lan, Suzane Kioko Ono-Nita,
Hideo Yoshida, Yasushi Shiratori, and Masao Omata

Introduction

Hepatitis C virus (HCV) is a positive-stranded RNA virus of genomic size of approximately 10 kilobases which is distantly related to the flaviviruses and the pestiviruses of the flavivirus family [1,2]. HCV RNA is detected in the serum of patients with non-A, non-B hepatitis using the assay method of reverse transcription followed by the polymerase chain reaction (RT-PCR). RT-PCR analysis of HCV RNA shows that the majority of anti-HCV-positive patients with chronic liver disease are HCV carriers [3]. The HCV genome contains a large open reading frame encoding a polyprotein precursor of 3010–3033 amino acids and an untranslated region (UTR) at the 5′ and 3′ ends of the genome. The putative organization of the HCV genome includes the 5′ UTR, 3 structural proteins, 7 nonstructural (NS) proteins, and the 3′ UTR, in order from the 5′ end [4]. One of the NS proteins, NS5A protein, is a serine phosphoprotein with two isoforms, p56 and p58 (the hyperphosphorylated form of p56) [5]. Clinically, a close association was demonstrated between mutations in the NS5A gene of HCV-1b and the response to interferon-α in patients with chronic active hepatitis [6,7]. Recently, the NS5A protein was shown to bind interferon-induced antiviral protein, PKR (double-stranded RNA-dependent protein kinase), and inhibit its kinase activity [8]. However, the function of the NS5A protein is still not fully understood. The NS5A protein was found to possess a nuclear localization-like signal sequence and to be localized in the nuclear periplasmic membrane fraction, so it seems that it may have some function related to transcription or translation [9].

Second Department of Internal Medicine, Faculty of Medicine, University of Tokyo, 7-3-1 Hongo, Bunkyo-ku, Tokyo 113-8655, Japan

In this study we show that amino-terminal (N-terminal) deleted-HCV NS5A protein fused with DNA-binding domain (DNA-BD) of GAL4, a yeast transcriptional activator, strongly activates transcription in yeast and mammalian cells (Huh7 human hepatoma cells) [10]. In addition, the transcriptional activation domain of the NS5A protein was analyzed using deletion mutants.

Materials and Methods

Construction of pGBT9-NS5A Plasmids

HCV RNA was extracted from the sera of patients with chronic hepatitis C type 1b using SepaGene-RV (Sankyo Junyaku, Tokyo, Japan). HCV genotyping was performed using PCR with type-specific primers [11]. The nucleotide sequences of the synthetic primers used in the RT-nested PCR are listed in Table 1. Part of the HCV NS5A region was amplified by

Table 1. PCR oligonucleotide primers used to construct the pGBT9-NS5A and pM-NS5A plasmids

Primer	Sequence[a]	Position[b]
Sense primer		
FK	5'-CTCTCCAGCCTTACCATCAC-3'	6171–6190
F5	5'-cgcggaTCCGCTCCGGCTCGTGGCTAAAGGA-3'	6246–6265
F10	5'-TGGATGGAGTGCGGTTGCACAGGTA-3'	6703–6727
F11	5'-cgcggatccCCGGCGTGCAGACCTCTCCT-3'	6732–6751
F14	5'-cgcggatccACAAGGTGGTGGTCCTAGACT-3'	7072–7092
F15	5'-cgcggatccGGACGGTTGTCCTGACAGAGTC-3'	7321–7342
F16	5'-cgcggatccCTTCAGCTAGCCAGTTGTCTG-3'	6931–6951
F18	5'-cgcggatcCGGGTGGGGGATTTCCACTA-3'	6612–6631
F19	5'-cgcggatcCATGTCAAAAACGGTTCCATGA-3'	6441–6462
F20	5'-cgcggatCCCCGAATTCTTCACGGAAT-3'	6683–6702
Antisense primer		
RK	5'-TCCTTGAGCACTGCCCGGTA-3'	7795–7776
R5	5'-cgcggatccGCAGCAGACGATGTCGTCGC-3'	7586–7567
R9	5'-cgcggatccCCTCTTTCTCCGTGGAGGTGG-3'	7322–7302
R13	5'-cgcggatccATTCTCTGACTCCACACGGGTGA-3'	7073–7051
R17	5'-cgcggatccAGAGTGGCCAAGGAGGGGG-3'	6932–6913

[a] Nucleotides complementary to the HCV genome are in *upper case*. *Bam*HI sites are *underlined*.
[b] The position is relative to the position in the prototype HCV type 1b, HCV-J [37].

RT-seminested PCR using primers F10 and R9 in the first PCR, and primers F11 and R9 in the second PCR. RT-PCR was performed as previously described [12]. Amplified products were digested with *Bam*HI and then cloned into the *Bam*HI site of pGBT9 (Clontech Laboratories, Palo Alto, CA, USA), a yeast expression vector, to generate a fused protein of NS5A and GAL4 DNA-BD. Cloned plasmids were purified using the Qiagen plasmid kit (Qiagen, Hilden, Germany). Nucleotide sequencing of the cloned plasmids, pGBT9-NS5A/UK1 and pGBT9-NS5A/UK2, from different patients with chronic hepatitis C type 1b, was performed using an autosequencer (PE Applied Biosystems, Foster City, CA, USA) and the dye-termination method, as described previously [13]. The amino acid sequences of the NS5A/UK1 and NS5A/UK2 segments were then compared using the computer software package Genetyx-Mac (Software Development, Tokyo, Japan).

Transformation of Yeast with pGBT9-NS5A and β-Galactosidase Assay

Experiments with yeast and mammalian cells were performed using the TransAct assay kit (Clontech). The yeast reporter strain used was Y187 (genotype: MATα, ura3-52, his3-200, ade2-101, *trp*1-901, *leu*2-3, 112, *gal*4Δ, *met*⁻, *gal*80Δ, URA3::GAL1$_{UAS}$-GAL1$_{TATA}$-*lacZ*) containing an integrated *lacZ* reporter construct which was regulated by the wild-type GAL1 promoter (Clontech). Yeast cells were made competent for transformation by treatment with lithium acetate as described previously [14]. pCL1 (Clontech), a yeast expression plasmid encoding the full-length wild-type GAL4, was used as a positive control, and pGBT9-HA (Clontech), a yeast expression plasmid encoding a DNA-BD/hemagglutinin epitope fusion protein, was used as a weak-positive control. Competent cells were transformed with pGBT9, pCL1, pGBT9-HA, pGBT9-NS5A/UK1, or pGBT9-NS5A/UK2. β-Galactosidase activity was determined using *o*-nitrophenyl β-D-galactopyranoside as the substrate as previously described [15]. Assays were performed in triplicate.

Construction of pM-NS5A Plasmids

HCV RNA was extracted from the serum of a 53-year-old male patient with HCV type 1b chronic active hepatitis as above. The full-length NS5A region was amplified by the long RT-nested PCR method using the LA RT-PCR kit (Takara Shuzo, Kyoto, Japan), with primers FK and RK for the first PCR and primers F5 and R5 for the second PCR. The amplified product was digested with *Bam*HI and then cloned into the *Bam*HI site of pM (Clontech), a mammalian expression vector, to generate a DNA-BD/ NS5A hybrid protein under the control of an SV40 promoter. Subsequent PCRs using pM-NS5A/F5-R5 (full-length NS5A-cloned pM) as the template were performed using primers of various NS5A regions to prepare various deletion mutants (Table 1). PCR products were digested with *Bam*HI and then cloned into the *Bam*HI site of pM. Nucleotide sequences of these plasmids were determined using an autosequencer.

Transfection of pM-NS5A into Huh7 Cells

Huh7 cells (Human Science Research Resource Bank, Osaka, Japan) were grown in RPMI 1640 supplemented with 0.5% fetal bovine serum (FBS) and 10% lactoalbumin at 37°C in 5% CO_2 atmosphere [16]. Approximately 1×10^6 Huh7 cells were plated onto 6-cm tissue culture plates (Iwaki Glass, Chiba, Japan) 24 h before transfection. Transfection of plasmids into Huh7 cells was performed using Lipofectamine (Life Technologies, Rockville, MD, USA). The efficiency of transfection was checked by cotransfection of the β-galactosidase expression plasmid pCMVβ (Clontech) with a series of pM-NS5A plasmids and pG5CAT (Clontech), a chloramphenicol acetyltransferase (CAT) reporter plasmid possessing five GAL4 binding sites and an adenovirus E1b minimum promoter upstream from the CAT gene. Briefly, transfection was carried out by adding to each tissue culture plate 3 ml Opti-MEM I reduced serum medium (Life Technologies) containing 2.5 μg pM-NS5A, 2.5 μg pG5CAT, 1 μg pCMVβ, and 24 μl Lipofectamine. pM3-VP16 (Clontech), a mammalian expression plasmid encoding the herpes virus protein VP16 fused with GAL4 DNA-BD, was used for positive control. After 16 h, 3 ml RPMI 1640 supplemented with 1% FBS and 20% lactoalbumin was added to each dish. After 24 h, the medium was changed to regular medium.

CAT Assay

Cells were harvested 48 h after transfection. CAT assays were carried out as described previously except that 1-deoxy[dichloroacetyl-1-^{14}C]chloramphenicol (Amersham International, Buckinghamshire, UK) was used as the substrate [15]. Assays were performed in triplicate. Autoradiography was performed and CAT activity was quantified using a

BAS2000 image analyzer (Fuji Photo Film, Tokyo, Japan) and normalized for transfection efficiency based on β-galactosidase activity.

Results

β-Galactosidase Assay of pGBT9-NS5A

pGBT9-NS5A/UK1 and pGBT9-NS5A/UK2 transformants exhibited marked β-galactosidase activity when assayed in liquid culture. β-Galactosidase units were calculated as described previously [17]. Data are shown in Table 2. The activities of pGBT9-NS5A/UK1 and pGBT9-NS5A/UK2 transformants were 90- and 25-times higher, respectively, than the activity of the pGBT9-HA transformant, the weak-positive control. Amino acid sequence analysis showed that the homology between the NS5A/UK1 segment and the NS5A/UK2 segment was 85% (168 amino acid residues were identical out of 197 amino acids) (Fig. 1).

CAT Assay of pM-NS5A

The N-terminal (146 amino acids (aa)) deletion mutants of the HCV NS5A protein fused with GAL4 DNA-BD (pM-NS5A/F20-R5) showed strong transcriptional activation, but the plasmid expressing the full-length HCV NS5A protein (pM-NS5A/F5-R5) showed no transcriptional activation (Fig. 2).

Of the N-terminal deletion mutants, pM-NS5A/F19-R5 (aa 2038–2419) and F18-R5 (aa 2095–2419) showed weak or no transcriptional activation, but the longer deletion mutants, F20-R5 (aa 2119–2419) and F11-R5 (aa

Table 2. β-Galactosidase activities of the pGBT9 plasmids

Plasmids	β-Galactosidase activity (units)	
	Mean	SD
pGBT9	0.1	0.05
pGBT9-HA	0.2	0.03
pCL	338	59
pGBT9-NS5A/UK1	18	3
pGBT9-NS5A/UK2	5	1

```
    2135
UK1 PVCKPLLREEVTFQVGLNQYLVGSQLPCEPEPDVAVLTSMLTDPSHITAETAKRRLARGS
UK2 ..................................................V....D........

    2195
UK1 PPSLGSSSASQLSAPSLKATCTTHHDSPDADLIEANLLWRQEMGGNITRVESENKVVILD
UK2 ....A....N..............L...LGV.........QH.........G..........

    2255
UK1 SFDPLRAEEDEREPSIPAEILRKSKKFPRALPIWASPEYNPPMLEPWKNPDYTPPVVHGC
UK2 ..E...........V.VA.......R...V.M.A..H.D....L....RD...V.......

    2315
UK1 PLATTKAPPIPPPRRKR
UK2 ..PPI.T..........
```

Fig. 1. Amino acid sequences of the NS5A/UK1 segment and NS5A/UK2 segment. *Numbers* represent the amino acid position of the prototype hepatitis C virus (*HCV*) type 1b, HCV-J [37]. Two acidic regions are *underlined*; a proline-rich region is *double-underlined*

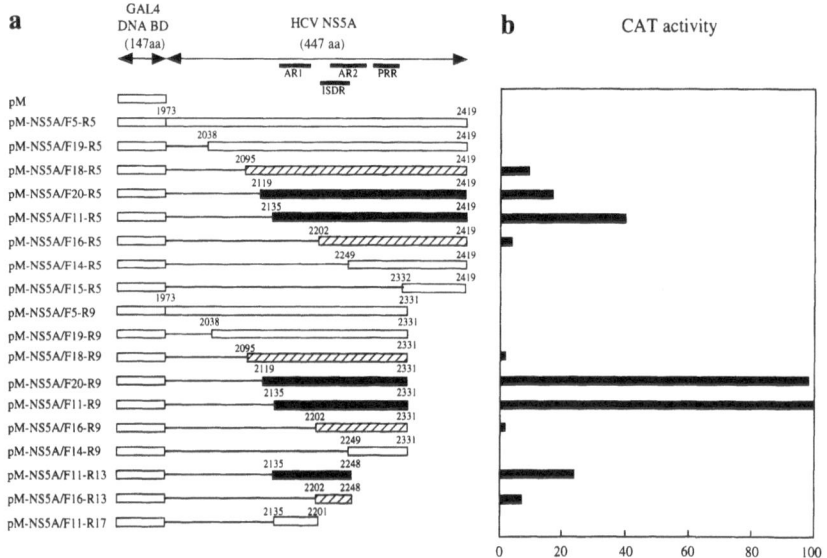

Fig. 2a,b. Identification of the HCV NS5A segment responsible for transcriptional activation. **a** *Bars* represent the segments of the HCV NS5A protein which are present. *Solid bars, hatched bars,* and *open bars* indicate the HCV NS5A protein mutants that activate transcription strongly, poorly, or not at all, respectively. *Numbers* indicate the amino acid position in the prototype HCV type 1b, HCV-J [37]. *AR1*, acidic region 1; *AR2*, acidic region 2; *PRR*, proline-rich region; *ISDR*, interferon sensitivity determining region. **b** Chloramphenicol acetyltransferase (*CAT*) activity was normalized by taking the highest activity (pM-NS5A/F11-R9) as 100. Results are expressed as the mean of three experiments, shown by *solid bars*

2135–2419), showed strong transcriptional activation, and the even longer deletion mutants, F16-R5 (aa 2202–2419), F14-R5 (aa 2249–2419), and F15-R5 (aa 2332–2419), showed weak or no transcriptional activation. The carboxy-terminal (C-terminal) (88 amino acids) deletion mutants showed a similar pattern as the N-terminal deletion mutants. That is, of these C-terminal deletion mutants, pM-NS5A/F5-R9 (aa 1973–2331), F19-R9 (aa 2038–2331) and F18-R9 (aa 2095–2331) showed little or no activity, but F20-R9 (aa 2119–2331) and F11-R9 (aa 2135–2331) activated transcription strongly, and F16-R9 (aa 2202–2331) and F14-R9 (aa 2249–2331) showed weak or no transcriptional activation. The longer deletion mutants, pM-NS5A/F11-R13 (aa 2135–2248) still showed distinct transcriptional activation, while F11-R17 (aa 2135–2201), the N-terminal part of F11-R13, and F16-R13 (aa 2202–2248), the C-terminal part of F11-R13, showed weak or no transcriptional activation. Expression of the fusion proteins was examined by Western blot using soluble protein cell extracts and monoclonal antibody against GAL4 DNA-BD (Clontech) following standard Western blotting procedures (data not shown) [18].

Analysis of the NS5A protein deletion mutants revealed that the domain of transcriptional activation may exist within the F11-R9 segment of the HCV NS5A protein (aa 2135–2331), because other deletion mutants (pM-NS5A/F16-R9, F14-R9, F11-R13, F16-R13, and F11-R17), which have longer deletions, showed weak or no transcriptional activation. A representative result of the CAT assay is shown in Fig. 3. The nucleotide sequence of the F11-R9 segment was confirmed bidirectionally and then deduced into-amino acids (Fig. 4). The net charge of 30 sequential amino acids was measured at 5-amino-acid intervals (see Fig. 5 for charge distribution within the NS5A/F11-R9 segment). Analysis of the amino acid sequence of the F11-R9 segment revealed that the purported transcriptional activation domain contained two acidic regions (AR1 and AR2) and one proline-rich region (PRR). The HCV NS5A/F11-R9 segment showed no homology with previously reported amino acid sequences as analyzed using the Genetyx-Mac/CD computer software package.

Discussion

The NS5A protein is a serine phosphoprotein with two isoforms, p56 and p58. The p58 isoform is a hyperphosphorylated form of p56, and its presence depends on the presence of NS4A protein [5]. The NS5A protein possesses a nuclear localization-like signal sequence and is present in the

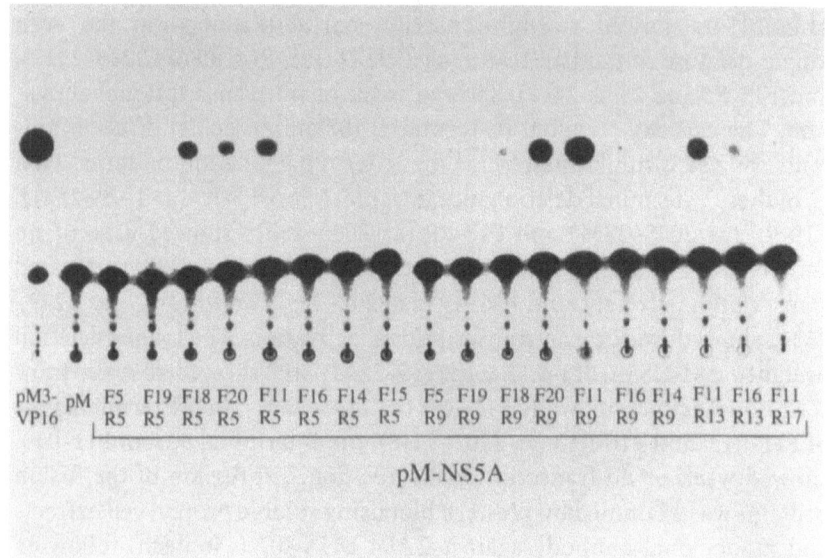

Fig. 3. Representative CAT assay of transcriptional activation by pM-NS5A. *pM3-VP16* was used as the positive control; *VP16* is a herpes virus protein which is a strong transcriptional activator. *pM* is a wild-type plasmid used as the negative control

```
2135          2145         2155         2165         2175         2185
  +      +--                      -    --            -           +++  +
PACRPLLRDE VTFQVGLNQY PVGSQLPCEP EPDVTVITSM LTDPSHITAE AAKRRLARGS

2195          2205         2215         2225         2235         2245
                          +          -   -  --  -    +  -        +    --- -        -
PPSLASSSAS QLSAPSLKAT CTTWHDSPDA DLIEANLLWR QEMGGNITRV ESENEVVVLD

2255          2265         2275         2285         2295         2305
  -   +  ---   -+-      -     ++ ++  .          .  +.       ..    +.       ..
SFEPLRAEED EREVSVAAEI LRKTRRFPAA MPVWARPDYN PPLLESWKNP XYVPPVVHGC

2315          2325
 . .. +  ..    ...+++++
PLPPTRAPPI PPPRRKR
```

Fig. 4. Amino acid sequence of the F11-R9 segment of the HCV NS5A protein. *Numbers* represent the amino acid position in the prototype HCV type 1b, HCV-J [37]. Positively charged residues (*R* and *K*) are marked + and negatively charged residues (*D* and *E*) are marked −. The two acidic regions are *underlined* and the proline-rich region is *double-underlined*. Proline residues in the PRR are *dotted*

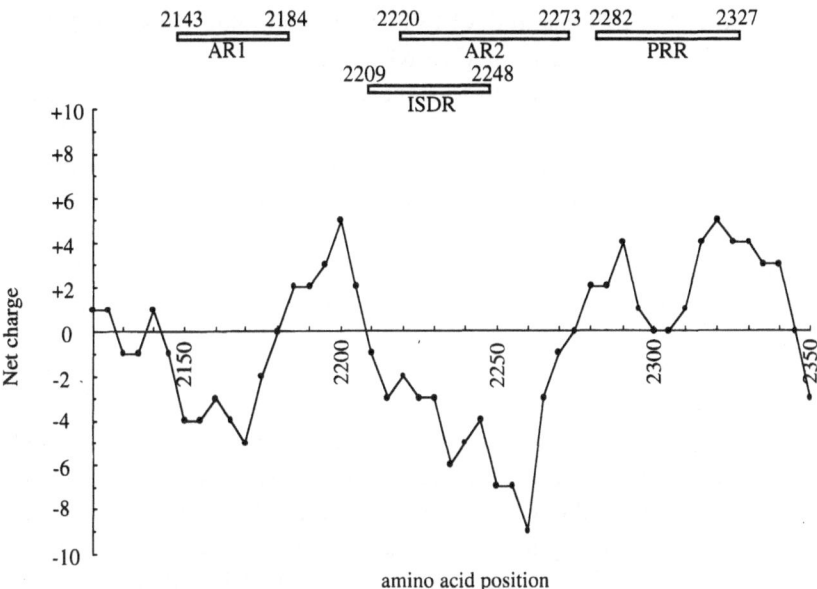

Fig. 5. Purported functional regions and charge distribution within the F11-R9 segment of the HCV NS5A protein. Shown is the net charge of 30 sequential-amino-acids measured at 5 amino acid intervals. *Numbers* indicate the amino acid position in the prototype HCV type 1b, HCV-J [37]. *AR1*, acidic region 1; *AR2*, acidic region 2; *PRR*, proline-rich region; *ISDR*, interferon sensitivity determining region

nuclear periplasmic membrane fraction, which indicates that it may have some function related to transcription or translation [9]; however, its function is still unknown. We have found that the NS5A protein deleted of its 146 N-terminal amino acids exhibited strong transcriptional activation. Analysis of various NS5A deletion mutants shows that the domain of transcriptional activation should exist within the F11-R9 segment (197 amino acids, from 2135 to 2331) of the HCV NS5A protein. This segment contains two acidic regions, AR1 and AR2, and one proline-rich region, PRR. AR1 consists of 42 amino acids (from 2143 to 2184 of the HCV NS5A region) with 7 acidic residues (Glu or Asp) (17%), and AR2 consists of 54 amino acids (from 2220 to 2273) with 16 acidic residues (Glu or Asp) (30%). PRR consists of 46 amino acids (from 2282 to 2327) with 16 proline residues (35%). These acidic and proline-rich domains in addition to a glutamine-rich domain are considered consensus motifs of a transcriptional activation domain [19–21]. As examples, an acidic domain exists in

GAL4 and GCN4 of yeast and VP16 of herpes simplex virus [22–24]. A proline-rich domain exists in CTF/NF1, Jun, AP2, and Oct2 [25]. Although the actual contribution to transcriptional activation of the AR1, AR2, and PRR domains is as yet unknown, their contribution seems to be cooperative since mutants with more extensive deletions showed weak or no transcriptional activation. AR1 and AR2 seem to be essential for transcriptional activation, and although PRR seems not to be essential for transcriptional activation it seems to enhance it, since the pM-NS5A/F11-R13 mutant, lacking the PRR of the pM-NS5A/F11-R9 mutant, showed distinct transcriptional activation.

The full-length HCV NS5A protein fused with GAL4 DNA-BD did not activate transcription. The 146 N-terminal amino acids may mask the function of transcriptional activation. It may be that the 146 N-terminal amino acids are a regulatory region. For example, HCV NS4A protein (p4) was found to bind to the N-terminal region of the NS5A protein, and the NS5A protein is hyperphosphorylated at serine residues in a NS4A-dependent manner [26]. Therefore, it may be possible that the NS4A protein functions as a regulatory factor. A similar phenomenon has been demonstrated for hMTF-1, a heavy metal-responsive transcription regulator in humans. Full-length hMTF-1 shows only weak transcriptional activation in the absence of heavy metals. The N-terminal part of hMTF-1 is a regulatory domain for metal induction. Therefore, hMTF-1 with the N-terminal region deleted shows transcriptional activation when fused to GAL4 DNA-BD [27].

Although the HCV NS5A protein is shown to be a potent transcriptional activator, its actual function is still not known. HCV is a causative agent of hepatocellular carcinoma which occurs all over the world, although the mechanism is still unknown [28–30]. It may be possible that the NS5A protein plays a role in hepatocarcinogenesis, since many other viral proteins that play a role in carcinogenesis often function as transcriptional activators. Actually, retrovirus oncogenes such as myc, fos, jun, myb, Rel, maf, and Ets are all DNA-binding transcriptional activators. The human T-cell leukemia virus type 1 oncogene Tax (transcriptional activator coded in the X-region) is also a transcriptional activator but it has no DNA-binding ability [31]. In fact, DNA virus oncogenes such as adenovirus early region 1A (E1A), simian virus 40 (SV40) large T antigen, and papillomavirus E6/E7 are transcriptional activators that have no DNA-binding ability [32–34]. Recently it was shown that NIH 3T3 mouse fibroblasts could be transformed with HCV NS3 cDNA and were then tumorigenic in nude mice [35]. Transformation of cells with the NS5A protein should be investigated with respect to oncogenic activity.

In a recent study, the amino acid residues 2209 to 2248 (interferon sensitivity determining region, ISDR) of the HCV-1b NS5A protein were implicated in responsiveness to interferon-α therapy in patients with chronic active hepatitis and serum HCV RNA level [6,7]. The NS5A F11-R9 segment (aa 2135–2419) contains the ISDR (aa 2209–2248). Thus, it may be that the NS5A protein affects response to interferon and viral replication through the function of transcriptional activation by regulating the transcription of certain cellular factors that have antiviral function or play a role in replication. Mutations in this region affected transcription in yeast (Table 1 and Fig. 1) as well as in Huh7 cells (unpublished data). Sequence analysis of many strains of HCV revealed that there is a high degree of interstrain as well as intrastrain nonhomology, which suggests that different strains with different capacities for transcriptional activation may be a reason for the clinical differences between patients infected with different strains of HCV [36].

The results of this study clearly show that the HCV NS5A protein is a potent transcriptional activator. However, its DNA-binding ability, cellular target, and the relationship between its activity and state of phosphorylation are still not known. Further investigations are necessary to elucidate the functions of this protein.

References

1. Choo Q-L, Kuo G, Weiner AJ, Overby LR, Bradley DW, Houghton M (1989) Isolation of a cDNA clone derived from a blood-borne non-A, non-B viral hepatitis genome. Science 244:359–362
2. Miller RH, Purcell RH (1990) Hepatitis C virus shares amino acid sequence similarity with pestiviruses and flaviviruses as well as members of two plant virus supergroups. Proc Natl Acad Sci USA 87:2057–2061
3. Kato N, Yokosuka O, Omata M, Hosoda K, Ohto M (1990) Detection of hepatitis C virus ribonucleic acid in the serum by amplification with polymerase chain reaction. J Clin Invest 86:1764–1767
4. Choo Q-L, Richman KH, Han JH, Berger K, Lee C, Dong C, Gallegos C, Coito D, Medina-Selby R, Barr PJ, Weiner AJ, Bradley DW, Kuo G, Houghton M (1991) Genetic organization and diversity of the hepatitis C virus. Proc Natl Acad Sci USA 88:2451–2455
5. Kaneko T, Tanji Y, Satoh S, Hijikata M, Asabe S, Kimura K, Shimotohno K (1994) Production of two phosphoproteins from the NS5A region of the hepatitis C virus genome. Biophys Biochem Res Commun 205:320–326

6. Enomoto N, Sakuma I, Asahina Y, Kurosaki M, Murakami T, Yamamoto C, Izumi N, Marumo F, Sato C (1995) Comparison of full-length sequences of interferon-sensitive and resistant hepatitis C virus 1b: sensitivity to interferon is conferred by amino acid substitutions in the NS5A region. J Clin Invest 96:224–230

7. Enomoto N, Sakuma I, Asahina Y, Kurosaki M, Murakami T, Yamamoto C, Ogura Y, Izumi N, Marumo F, Sato C (1996) Mutations in the nonstructural protein 5A gene and response to interferon in patients with chronic hepatitis C virus 1b infection. N Engl J Med 334:77–81

8. Gale MJ Jr, Korth MJ, Tang NM, Tan S-L, Hopkins DA, Dever TE, Polyak SJ, Gretch DR, Katze MG (1997) Evidence that hepatitis C virus resistant to interferon is mediated through repression of the PKR protein kinase by the nonstructural 5A protein. Virology 230:217–227

9. Tanji Y, Kaneko T, Satoh S, Shimotohno K (1995) Phosphorylation of hepatitis C virus-encoded nonstructural protein NS5A. J Virol 69:3980–3986

10. Kato N, Lan K-H, Ono-Nita SK, Shiratori Y, Omata M (1997) Hepatitis C virus nonstructural region 5A protein is a potent transcriptional activator. J Virol 71:8856–8859

11. Okamoto H, Sugiyama Y, Okada S, Kurai K, Akahane Y, Sugai Y, Tanaka T, Sato K, Tsuda F, Miyakawa Y, Mayumi M (1992) Typing hepatitis C virus by polymerase chain reaction with type-specific primers: application to clinical surveys and tracing infectious sources. J Gen Virol 73:673–679

12. Kato N, Yokosuka O, Hosoda K, Ito Y, Ohto M, Omata M (1993) Detection of hepatitis C virus RNA in acute non-A, non-B hepatitis as an early diagnostic tool. Biochem Biophys Res Commun 192:800–807

13. Togo G, Toda N, Kanai F, Kato N, Shiratori Y, Kishi K, Imazeki F, Makuuchi M, Omata M (1996) A transforming growth factor β type II receptor gene mutation common in sporadic cecum cancer with microsatellite instability. Cancer Res 56:5620–5623

14. Becker DM, Guarente L (1991) High-efficiency transformation of yeast by electroporation. In: Guthrie C, Fink GR (eds) Methods in enzymology, vol. 194, Guide to yeast genetics and molecular biology. Academic, San Diego, pp 182–187

15. Sambrook J, Fritsch EF, Maniatis T (1989) Expression of cloned genes in cultured mammalian cells. In: Nolan C (ed) Molecular cloning, a laboratory manual, 2nd edn. Cold Spring Harbor Laboratory, Plainview, pp 16.1–16.81

16. Nakabayashi H, Taketa K, Miyano K, Yamane T, Sato J (1982) Growth of human hepatoma cells lines with differentiated functions in chemically defined medium. Cancer Res 42:3858–3863

17. Miller JH (1972) Experiments in molecular genetics. Cold Spring Harbor Laboratory, Cold Spring Harbor

18. Sambrook J, Fritsch EF, Maniatis T (1989) Detection and analysis of proteins expressed from cloned genes. In: Nolan C (ed) Molecular cloning, a laboratory manual, 2nd edn. Cold Spring Harbor Laboratory, Plainview, pp 18.1–18.88

19. Courey AJ, Tjian R (1988) Analysis of Sp1 in vivo reveals multiple transcriptional domains, including a novel glutamine-rich activation motif. Cell 55:887–898

20. Ma J, Ptashne M (1987) A new class of yeast transcriptional activators. Cell 51:113–119
21. Mermod N, O'Neill EA, Kelly TJ, Tjian R (1989) The proline-rich transcriptional activator of CTF/NF-1 is distinct from the replication and DNA binding domain. Cell 58:741–753
22. Campbell ME, Palfreyman JW, Preston CM (1984) Identification of herpes simplex virus DNA sequences which encode a trans-acting polypeptide responsible for stimulation of immediate early transcription. J Mol Biol 180:1–19
23. Hope IA, Struhl K (1986) Functional dissection of a eukaryotic transcriptional activator protein, GCN4 of yeast. Cell 46:885–894
24. Ma J, Ptashne M (1987) Deletion analysis of GAL4 defines two transcriptional activating segments. Cell 48:847–853
25. Mitchell PJ, Tjian R (1989) Transcriptional regulation in mammalian cells by sequence-specific DNA binding proteins. Science 245:371–378
26. Asabe S, Tanji Y, Satoh S, Kaneko T, Kimura K, Shimotohno K (1997) The N-terminal region of hepatitis C virus-encoded NS5A is important for NS4A-dependent phosphorylation. J Virol 71:790–796
27. Radtke F, Georgiev O, Muller H-P, Brugnera E, Schaffner W (1995) Functional domains of the heavy metal-responsive transcription regulator MTF-1. Nucleic Acids Res 23:2277–2286
28. Kuo G, Choo Q-L, Alter HJ, Gitnick GL, Redeker AG, Purcell RH, Miyamura T, Dienstag JL, Alter MJ, Stevens CE, Tegtmeier GE, Bonino F, Colombo M, Lee AS, Kuo C, Berger K, Shuster JR, Overby LR, Bradley DW, Houghton M (1989) An assay for circulating antibodies to a major etiologic virus of human non-A, non-B hepatitis. Science 344:362–364
29. Okuda K (1992) Hepatocellular carcinoma: recent progress. Hepatology 15:948–963
30. Saito I, Miyamura T, Ohbayashi A, Harada H, Katayama T, Kikuchi S, Watanabe Y, Koi S, Onji M, Ohta Y, Choo Q-L, Houghton M, Kuo G (1990) Hepatitis C virus infection is associated with the development of hepatocellular carcinoma. Proc Natl Acad Sci USA 87:6547–6549
31. Seiki M, Inoue J, Takeda T, Yoshida M (1986) Direct evidence that p40x of human T-cell leukemia virus type I is a trans-acting transcriptional activator. EMBO J 5:561–565
32. Berk AJ (1986) Adenovirus promoters and E1A transactivation. Annu Rev Genet 20:45–79
33. Manfredi JJ, Prives C (1994) The transforming activity of simian virus 40 large tumor antigen. Biochim Biophys Acta 1198:65–83
34. Schwarz E, Freese UK, Gissmann L, Mayer W, Roggenbuck A, Stremlau B, zur Hausen H (1985) Structure and transcription of human papillomavirus sequences in cervical carcinoma cells. Nature 314:111–114
35. Sakamuro D, Furukawa T, Takegami T (1995) Hepatitis C virus nonstructural protein NS3 transforms NIH 3T3 cells. J Virol 69:3893–3896
36. Kato N, Shiratori Y, Omata M (1996) Hepatitis C virus genotypes: molecular basis and clinical significance. In: Boyer JL, Ockner RK (eds) Progress in liver diseases, vol. XIV. Saunders, Philadelphia, pp 223–244

37. Kato N, Hijikata M, Ootsuyama Y, Nakagawa N, Ohkoshi S, Sugimura T, Shimotohno K (1990) Molecular cloning of the human hepatitis C virus genome from Japanese patients with non-A, non-B hepatitis. Proc Natl Acad Sci USA 87:9524–9528

Natural Variation in Translational Activities of the 5' Nontranslated RNAs of Genotypes 1a and 1b Hepatitis C Virus: Evidence for a Long Range RNA–RNA Interaction Outside of the Internal Ribosomal Entry Segment

Masao Honda[1], Geoff Abell[2], Shuichi Kaneko[1],
Kenichi Kobayashi[1] and Stanley M. Lemon[2]

Introduction

Hepatitis C virus (HCV) is a positive-stranded, enveloped RNA virus which is classified within the hepacivirus genus of the family Flaviviridae [1]. There is extensive genetic heterogeneity among different HCV strains, with at least six major genotypes and a series of related subtypes recognized thus far [2,3]. Among these, genotype 1 is predominant worldwide and comprised of two major subtypes, genotypes 1a and 1b [2]. Although some clinical studies have found no differences in the clinical expression of liver disease that are related to the genotype of the infecting virus [4], others have suggested that genotype 1b infections may be more resistant to interferon therapy [5,6], and may confer greater risk for development of hepatocellular carcinoma than infection with nongenotype 1b strains including genotype 1a viruses [7].

We noted previously that the 5' nontranslated RNA (5'NTR) of a genotype 1a virus (Hutchinson strain, or HCV-H) directed translation with greater efficiency than that of a genotype 1b virus (HCV-H) when placed in the context of nearly genomic-length viral RNA [8]. We found the internal ribosomal entry sequence (IRES) of the genotype 1a virus to be about twofold more active than the genotype 1b virus, both in a cell-free translation system and in transfected Huh-T7 cells in vivo [8]. The sequences of the HCV-H and HCV-N 5'NTRs differ at only seven base positions, grouped at four locations within the 5'NTR (Fig. 1).

[1] First Department of Internal Medicine, Kanazawa University, 13-1 Takara-machi, Kanazawa 920-8640, Japan
[2] Departments of Microbiology and Immunology, The University of Texas Medical Branch at Galveston, Galveston, TX, 77555-1019, USA

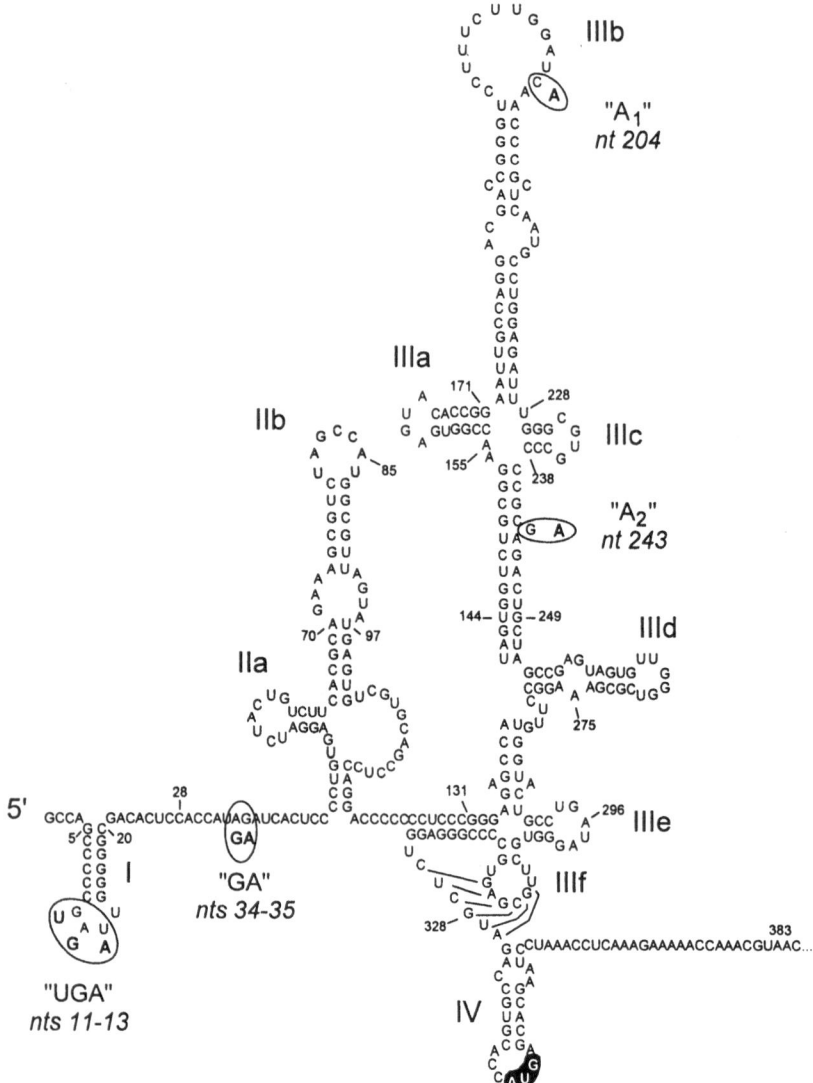

Fig. 1. Proposed secondary and tertiary RNA structures within the 5' nontranslated RNA (5'NTR) and the immediately downstream segment of the long open reading frame of the genotype 1b hepatitis C virus (HCV)-N virus. The *circled* nucleotides indicate differences between the sequences of HCV-N and the genotype 1a HCV-H virus, which are clustered into four groups: *UGA, GA, A_1,* and *A_2*

Here, we report that the difference in the translational activities of these two viruses is due to the presence of a AG dinucleotide sequence located at nucleotides (nts) 34–35 of the genotype 1b 5'NTR. This dinucleotide sequence is GA in the translationally more active genotype 1a 5'NTR. Although the AG dinucleotide sequence is upstream of the minimal essential IRES, it nonetheless exerts an inhibitory effect on IRES activity. However, this inhibitory effect is observed only when the 5'NTR is fused in its natural context to the HCV open reading frame. These results suggest the existence of a previously unrecognized interaction between RNA located upstream of the IRES, and a distant downstream sequence within the capsid coding region.

Results

HCV-H and HCV-N Translation in Rabbit Reticulocyte Lysate

To better quantify the difference in translational activities of the IRESs of HCV-N and HCV-H, we examined the ability of RNAs transcribed from pN-CΔE1 and pH-CΔE1 to direct translation of HCV proteins in rabbit reticulocyte lysate. These transcripts contain the 5'NTR sequences of HCV-N and HCV-H, respectively, fused naturally to nts 342–1357 of the open reading frame of HCV-N virus (Fig. 2a). The in vitro translation reactions (25 μl each) were programmed with 0.25–2 μg RNA (10–80 μg/μl), and supplemented with microsomal membranes to allow signalase cleavage at the capsid–E1 junction. The major products of translation included the 21 kDa capsid protein, a 30 kDa truncated, glycosylated E1 protein (ΔE1), and a 34 kDa unprocessed precursor protein (C-ΔE1) (Fig. 2b). At each RNA concentration, greater quantities of all of these proteins were produced by the HCV-H transcripts (Fig. 2b). On average, pH-CΔE1 transcripts produced a 2.4-fold greater quantity of the capsid protein and 1.8-fold greater quantity of ΔE1, compared with pN-CΔE1 transcripts.

Genetic Basis of the Difference in Translational Activities of Genotype 1a (HCV-H) and Genotype 1b (HCV-N) 5'NTRs

The 5'NTR sequences of the HCV-H and HCV-N viruses differ at seven nucleotide positions. These are grouped at four locations within the 5'NTR: nts 11–13, 34–35, 204, and 243 (Fig. 1). To determine which of these differences in the nucleotide sequences of the 5'NTRs were respon-

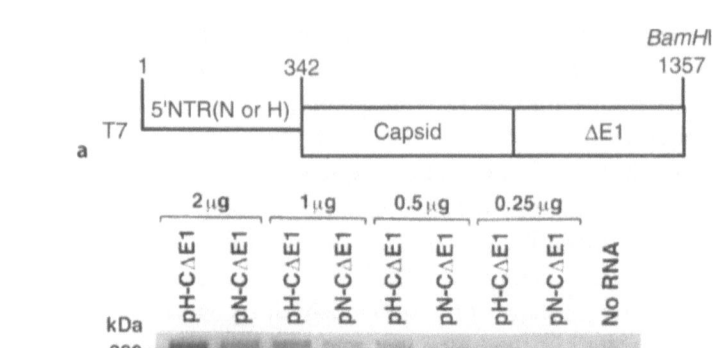

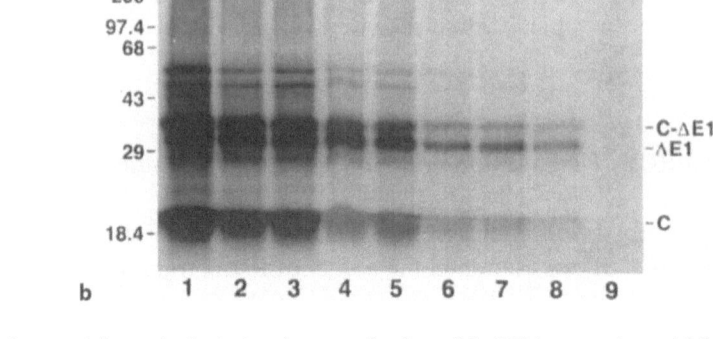

Fig. 2. a Schematic depicting the organization of the RNA transcripts which were used to program reticulocyte lysate for translation. The *solid line* depicts nontranslated RNA, while the sequence encoding the HCV proteins expressed by these transcripts is represented by the *open box*. **b** SDS-PAGE of products of translation from rabbit reticulocyte lysate programmed with 2 (*lanes 1 and 2*), 1 (*lanes 3 and 4*), 0.5 (*lanes 5 and 6*), 0.25 (*lanes 6 and 8*), or 0 (*lane 9*) µg RNA derived from pH-CΔE1 (containing the 5′NTR of HCV-H, *lanes 1, 3, 5, and 7*) or pN-CΔE1 (containing the 5′NTR of HCV-N, *lanes 2, 4, 6, and 8*) per 25 µl reaction

sible for the difference in translational activity, we constructed a series of chimeric 5′NTR constructs in which the four nucleotide substitution groups present in the HCV-H sequence (Fig. 1) were systematically introduced into the background of the HCV-N sequence in pN-CΔE1 (Fig. 3a). Plasmids pN-UGA, pN-GA, pN-A$_1$, and pN-A$_2$ contain the HCV-H substitutions at nts 11–13 (GAU → UGA), nts 34–35 (AG → GA), nt 204 (C → A), and nt 243 (G → A), respectively. The amounts of capsid and ΔE1 proteins produced from pN-GA transcripts (Fig. 3b, lane 4) were nearly equivalent to those produced by pH-CΔE1 transcripts (lane 2), while pN-UGA, pN-A$_1$, and pN-A$_2$ transcripts (lanes 3, 5, and 6) had translational activities approximating RNA transcribed from pN-CΔE1

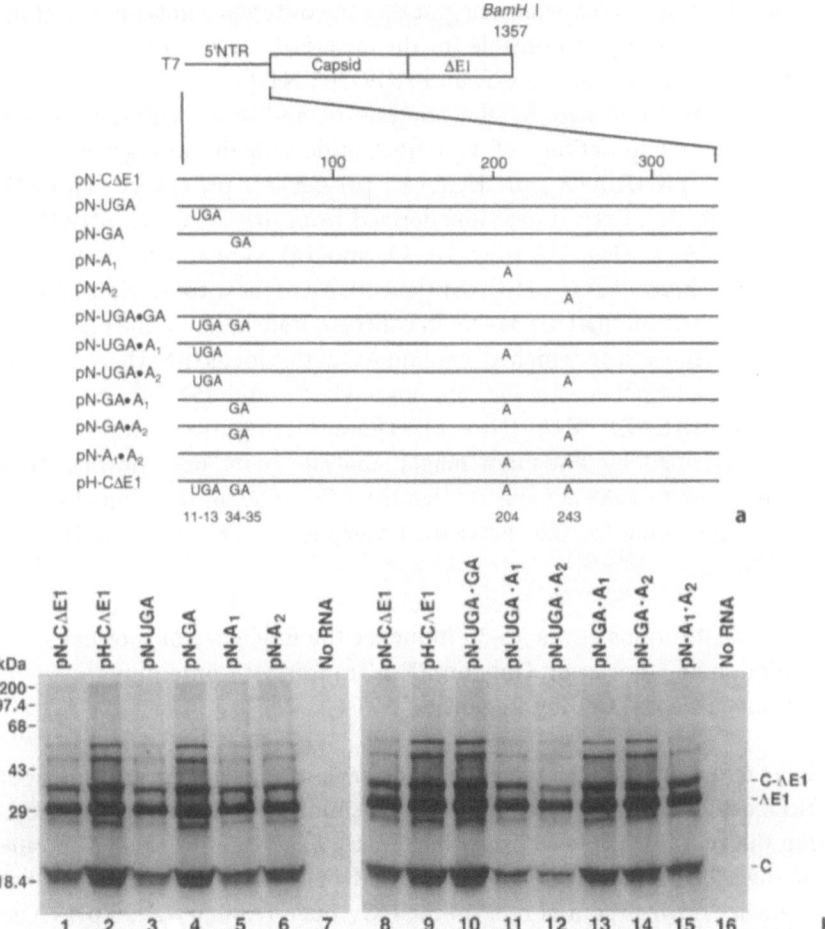

Fig. 3. a Organization of T7 transcriptional units within chimeric constructs containing the unique nucleotide sequences of HCV-H placed individually and in combination within the background of the HCV-N 5′NTR and immediately downstream segment of the open reading frame encoding CΔE1 (*pN-CΔE1*). Protein coding regions are shown as *rectangles*, while noncoding RNA is shown as a *solid line*. The map positions of the base substitutions are shown at the bottom of the figure. **b** SDS-PAGE of products of translation from reticulocyte lysate programmed with RNAs transcribed from the plasmids depicted in a. The two panels represent results from separate experiments. The gel positions of the capsid (*C*), *ΔE1*, and nonprocessed *C-ΔE1* protein products are shown at the right

(lane 1). Thus, these results suggest that the difference in sequence at nts 34–35 is primarily responsible for the observed variation in the translational activities of the HCV-H and HCV-N 5'NTRs.

This was confirmed by the analysis of additional chimeras which contained combinations of two nucleotide substitution groups: pN-UGA·GA, pN-UGA·A$_1$, pN-UGA·A$_2$, pN-GA·A$_1$, pN-GA·A$_2$, and pN-A$_1$·A$_2$ (Fig. 3a). RNA transcripts derived from pN-UGA·GA, pN-GA·A$_1$ and pN-GA·A$_2$ (Fig. 3b, lanes 10, 13, and 14) were translated with an efficiency equivalent to pH-CΔE1 (lane 9). All of these transcripts contain the GA substitution at nts 34–35. In contrast, translation of the remaining chimeric transcripts, which all contain AG at this locus (pN-UGA·A$_1$, pN-UGA·A$_2$, and pN-A$_1$·A$_2$, Fig. 3b, lanes 11, 12, and 15) did not exceed that of pN-CΔE1 RNA (lane 8). These findings were reproducible and confirmed by PhosphorImager analysis (data not shown). They strongly support the conclusion that the AG → GA substitution at nt 34–35 is responsible for the increased translational activity of the HCV-H 5'NTR.

Base Substitutions at nts 34–35 Influence the Efficiency of Internal Initiation of Translation Only on RNA Transcripts Containing the Complete Capsid Coding Region

In an effort to develop a sensitive reporter assay allowing measurement of IRES activity in vivo, we constructed plasmids in which sequence encoding the reporter protein, firefly luciferase, was fused in-frame at nt 408 of the HCV sequence in pN-CΔE1 and pH-CΔE1, thus replacing the sequence downstream of nt 66 of the HCV open reading frame (pN-CLuc and pH-CLuc, Fig. 4a). We also constructed dicistronic variants of these plasmids, in which sequence encoding CAT was placed upstream of the HCV 5'NTR (pCAT-N-CLuc and pCAT-H-CLuc, Fig. 4a). Surprisingly, we found that the type of 5'NTR sequence (HCV-H or HCV-N) had no influence on the translational efficiency of either the monocistronic (Fig. 4b, lane 1 vs 2) or dicistronic transcripts (lane 3 vs 4).

In contrast to these results, dicistronic transcripts in which the truncated HCV open reading frame (CΔE1) represented the downstream cistron (pCAT-N-CΔE1 and pCAT-H-CΔE1, Fig. 4a) retained the increased translational activity observed with the HCV-H 5'NTR in earlier analyses of monocistonic transcripts containing only HCV sequence (Figs. 2 and 3). The greater translational activity of the HCV-H 5'NTR was evident

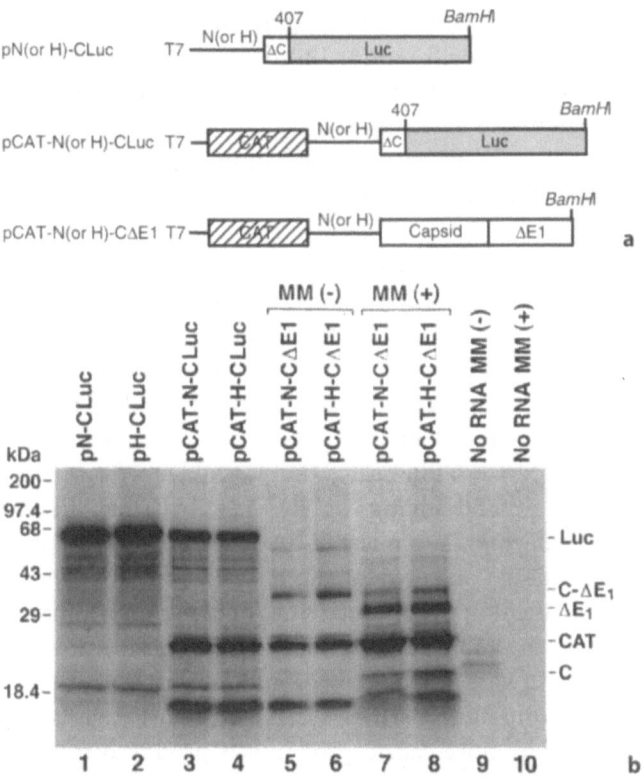

Fig. 4. a Organization of mono- and dicistronic T7 transcriptional units within the indicated plasmids. Protein coding regions are shown as *rectangles*, while noncoding RNA is shown as a *solid line*. The downstream cistrons are under translational control of the HCV 5′NTR, and contain the luciferase reporter protein-coding sequence (*Luc*) fused to nt 407 of the HCV sequence (codon 22 of the open reading frame), or the natural HCV-N sequence extending to nt 1357. The upstream cistron in the dicistronic plasmids encodes the bacterial enzyme, chloramphenicol acetyltransferase (*CAT*). **b** SDS-PAGE of products of translation from reticulocyte lysate programmed with monocistronic (*left panel*) or dicistronic (*right panel*) RNAs transcribed from the plasmids depicted in a. In *lanes 7, 8, and 10*, reactions were supplemented with microsomal membranes [*MM(+)*] while reactions in *lanes 1–6 and 9* did not contain membranes [*MM(−)*]. The gel positions of the capsid (*C*), ΔE1, nonprocessed *C-ΔE1*, luciferase, and CAT protein products are shown at the right

whether these reaction mixes were supplemented (Fig. 4b, lane 7 vs 8) or not supplemented (lane 5 vs 6) with microsomal membranes. Thus, although the base substitutions at nts 34–35 of the HCV-H 5'NTR are primarily responsible for its greater translational activity, the difference in translational activity that these substitutions confer is only evident when the translated sequence contains native HCV sequence downstream of nt 408.

To further define the downstream sequence required for the enhanced translational activity of the HCV-H 5'NTR, we compared nearly genomic-length dicistronic RNA transcripts containing the HCV-H or HCV-N 5'NTRs fused naturally to the HCV-N sequence extending to nt 9454 of the HCV genome (plasmids pCAT/N and pCAT/H) (Fig. 5a). While these RNAs produced equivalent amounts of CAT in reticulocyte lysate, PhosphorImager analyses indicated that 1.8-fold more capsid protein was produced from pCAT/H than pCAT/N (Fig. 5b). Thus, the inclusion of HCV sequence beyond the truncated CΔE1 segment did not influence the relative translational activities of the HCV-H and HCV-N 5'NTRs. We next examined the translational activities of dicistronic transcripts which contained only the capsid coding sequence within the downstream cistron. These RNAs were prepared by runoff transcription of MulI-digested pCAT-N-CΔE1 and pCAT-N-CΔE1, and PhosphorImager analyses indicated that 1.8-fold more capsid protein was produced from pCAT-H-C than from pCAT-N-C.

Expression of the Capsid Protein is Not Required for the Enhanced Translational Activity of HCV-H

The fact that we observed differences in the translational activities of the HCV-H and HCV-N 5'NTRs only when they were fused to the native HCV capsid sequence could be explained by differences in the interaction of these 5'NTRs with the capsid protein. Alternatively, the requirement for capsid sequence could reflect an interaction of this RNA with sequences within the 5'NTR. To distinguish between these two possibilities, we introduced frameshift mutations into the capsid coding sequence of pCAT-N-CΔE1 and pCAT-H-CΔE1. The resulting plasmids, pCAT-N-CΔE1(Fs) and pCAT-H-CΔE1(Fs) each contain two mutations: a -1 frameshift at nt 409 and a $+1$ frameshift at nt 769, the latter of which restores the original reading frame and maintains its patency to the end of the truncated E1 sequence (Fig. 6a). Thus, although transcripts produced

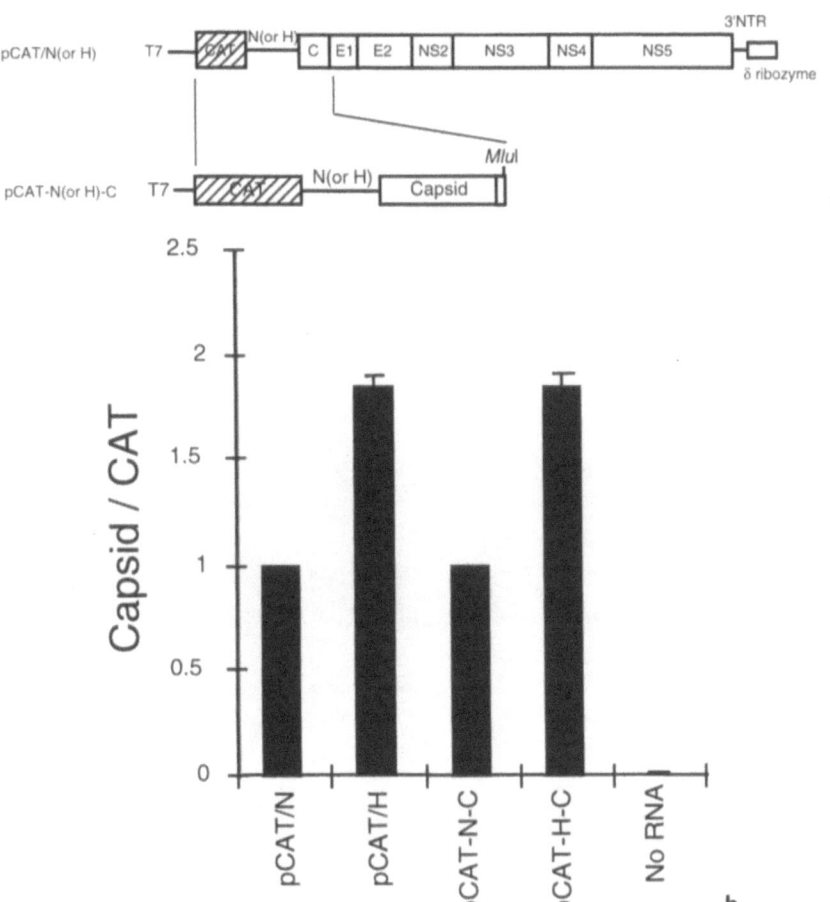

Fig. 5. a Organization of dicistronic T7 transcripts encoding CAT in the upstream cistron and HCV sequences in the downstream cistron, under translational control of the 5'NTRs of HCV-N or HCV-H. *pCAT/N* and *pCAT/H* contain the entire coding sequence of the HCV-N virus in addition to much of the 3'NTR. A hepatitis delta virus ribozyme sequence directs cleavage at the 3' terminus of the HCV sequences in these RNAs [11]. *pCAT-N-C* and *pCAT-H-C* contain only the capsid coding sequence and 15 nts of the E1 coding region, and were derived from runoff transcription. **b** PhosphorImager quantitation of the in vitro products of translation of the RNAs shown in **a**

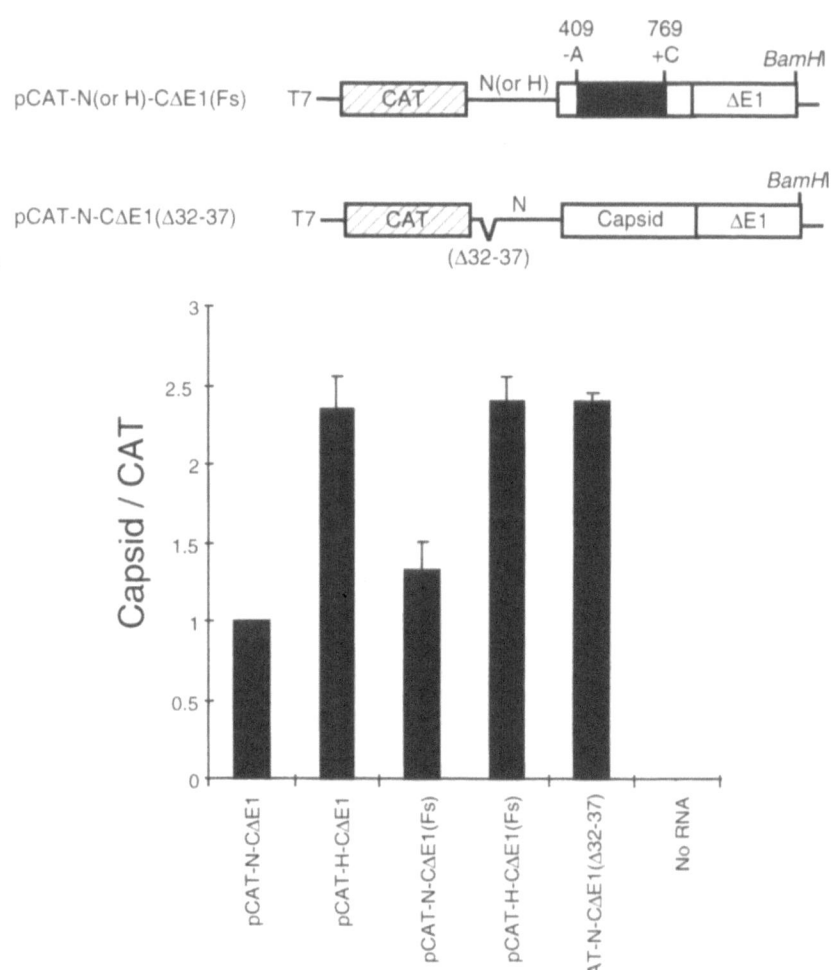

Fig. 6. a Organization of additional dicistronic T7 transcripts encoding CAT in the upstream cistron and HCV sequences in the downstream cistron. In *pCAT-N-CΔE1(Fs)* and *pCAT-H-CΔE1(Fs)* transcripts, the HCV capsid coding sequences contain −1 and +1 frame-shift mutations at nts 409 and 769, respectively, resulting in the expression of the C(Fs) protein which contains nonsense sequence (*solidly shaded segment*) replacing much of the natural capsid sequence. Nucleotides 32–37 are deleted from the HCV-N 5′NTR sequence within *pCAT-N-CΔE1 (Δ32–37)*. **b** PhosphorImager quantitation of the HCV capsid proteins produced in translation reactions similar to those shown in **a**

from these plasmids differ by only 2 nts from the RNAs transcribed from pCAT-N-CΔE1 and pCAT-H-CΔE1, they encode a markedly altered capsid protein, C(Fs), which consists of nonsense sequence between residues 23 and 143, or for approximately 63% of its sequence. The significantly greater quantities of these proteins were expressed from pCAT-H-CΔE1(Fs) compared with pCAT-N-CΔE1(Fs) transcripts (Fig. 6b). These data strongly suggest that the difference in IRES activity is dependent upon the nucleotide sequence of the RNA, and not the amino acid sequence of the protein which it encodes.

The AG Dinucleotide Sequence at nts 34–35 of HCV-N Has an Inhibitory Effect on IRES Function

Since the nature of the sequence at nts 34–35 was found to have such an important effect on the translational activity of HCV transcripts, it was of interest to further investigate whether the sequence in this region is required for the internal initiation of translation on these RNAs. We created a 6 nt deletion mutation (nts 32–37) in pCAT-N-CΔE1, resulting in the plasmid pCAT-N-CΔE1 (Δ32–37) (Fig. 6a). Interestingly, dicistronic transcripts derived from this plasmid retained robust IRES activity. The amount of capsid protein produced from the pCAT-N-CΔE1 (Δ32–37) transcripts (Fig. 6b) was approximately 2.4-fold higher than transcripts from pCAT-N-CΔE1, and approximately equivalent to transcripts containing the HCV-H 5′NTR. Thus, the sequence at nts 34–35 is not essential for IRES activity, and the presence of an AG dinucleotide at this position has an inhibitory effect on the activity of the IRES.

Discussion

Several studies suggest that genotype 1b infections may be relatively resistant to treatment with recombinant interferon-α [5,6], and perhaps are more likely to lead to development of hepatocellular carcinoma [7], despite the fact that levels of viremia appear to be equivalent in patients infected with either of these types of virus [9]. Preliminary data suggest that the proportion of patients infected with non-1b genotypes is increasing, largely because injection drug users are likely to be infected with genotypes 1a or 3a for unknown reasons [10]. Thus, it remains uncertain whether differences exist in the efficiency of virus transmission or pathogenicity among HCV strains of different genotypes.

We had noted previously that the 5'NTR of HCV-H, genotype 1a virus, was about twice as active as that of HCV-N, genotype 1b virus, in directing the internal initiation of translation of HCV RNA [8]. The present results indicate that this difference is due to the AG dinucleotide at nts 34–35 of the genotype 1b HCV-N virus (Fig. 3), which appears to suppress the activity of the downstream IRES when it is fused naturally to the HCV capsid coding sequence (Fig. 6). We found that the nucleotide sequence required for expression of the difference in translational activities lies between nts 408 and 929 of the HCV genome. The critical determinant is the RNA sequence, not the amino acid sequence of the protein which it encodes (Fig. 6). A further striking observation was that deletion of nts 32–37, including the AG dinucleotide sequence, from the HCV-N 5'NTR did not impair, but actually enhanced translation from dicistronic transcripts. The fact that RNA sequences within the coding region as well as upstream of the IRES act cooperatively to influence the activity of the IRES suggests that these upstream and downstream RNA segments physically interact with each other in a fashion that may influence the secondary or tertiary structure of RNA within the IRES.

We observed that the 5'NTR of HCV-H was approximately 2-fold more active than the 5'NTR of HCV-N in directing the translation of the capsid protein both. Could such a minimal difference in translational activity lead to differences in replication capacity and possibly the pathogenicity of these viruses? It is not possible to answer this question at present in the absence of cell culture systems which are permissive for HCV infection and which mimic the replicative environment of the hepatocyte in vivo. Other recent work in our laboratory has shown that mutations within the 5'NTR of hepatitis A virus which confer only a 4- to 6-fold increase in the internal initiation of translation by this picornavirus in monkey kidney cells result in a marked increase in the size of replication foci and in hepatitis A virus yields in these cells [11,12]. Thus, while there is no direct evidence that the 2-fold greater translational activity of the genotype 1a 5'NTR has a significant impact on viral replication or pathogenesis in vivo, this possibility cannot be excluded at present.

References

1. Choo Q-L, Kuo G, Weiner AJ, Overby LR, Bradley DW, Houghton M (1989) Isolation of a cDNA clone derived from a blood-borne non-A, non-B viral hepatitis genome. Science 244:359–362

2. Davidson F, Simmonds P, Ferguson JC, Jarvis LM, Dow BC, Follett EAC, Seed CRG, Krusius T, Lin C, Medgyesi GA, Kiyokawa H, Olim G, Duraisamy G, Cuypers T, Saeed AA, Teo D, Conradie J, Kew MC, Lin M, Nuchaprayoon C, Ndimbie OK, Yap PL (1995) Survey of major genotypes and subtypes of hepatitis C virus using RFLP of sequences amplified from the 5' non-coding region. J Gen Virol 76:1197–1204

3. Simmonds P, Holmes EC, Cha T-A, Chan S-W, McOmish F, Irvine B, Yap PL, Kolberg J, Urdea MS (1993) Classification of hepatitis C virus into six major genotypes and a series of subtypes by phylogenetic analysis of the NS-5 region. J Gen Virol 74:2391–2399

4. Lau JY, Davis GL, Prescott LE, Maertens G, Lindsay KL, Qian K, Mizokami M, Simmonds P, Hepatitis Interventional Therapy Group (1996) Distribution of hepatitis C virus genotypes determined by line probe assay in patients with chronic hepatitis C seen at tertiary referral centers in the United States. Ann Intern Med 124:868–876

5. Nousbaum J-B, Pol S, Nalpas B, Landais P, Berthelot P, Bréchot C, Collaborative Study Group (1995) Hepatitis C Virus type 1b (II) infection in France and Italy. Ann Intern Med 122:161–168

6. Zein NN, Persing DH (1996) Hepatitis C genotypes: current trends and future implications. Mayo Clin Proc 71:458–462

7. Silini E, Bottelli R, Asti M, Bruno S, Candusso ME, Brambilla S, Bono F, Iamoni G, Tinelli C, Mondelli MU, Ideo G (1996) Hepatitis C virus genotypes and risk of hepatocellular carcinoma in cirrhosis: A case-control study. Gastroenterology 111:199–205

8. Honda M, Ping L-H, Rijnbrand RCA, Amphlett E, Clarke B, Rowlands D, Lemon SM (1996) Structural requirements for initiation of translation by internal ribosomal entry within genome-length hepatitis C virus RNA. Virology 222:31–42

9. Smith DB, Davidson F, Yap PL, Brown H, Kolberg J, Detmer J, Urdea M, Simmonds P, Mellor J, Neville J, Prescott L, Dow BC, Follett EAC, Skuldamrongpanich T, Tanprasert S, Nuchaprayoon C, Lin CK, Kew MC, Crookes R, Conradie JD, Lin M, Seed C, De Olim GAB, Martins IA (1996) Levels of hepatitis C virus in blood donors infected with different viral genotypes. J Infect Dis 173:727–730

10. Pol S, Thiers V, Nousbaum J-B, Legendre C, Berthelot P, Kreis H, Brechot C (1995) The changing relative prevalence of hepatitis C virus genotypes: evidence in hemodialyzed patients and kidney recipients. Gastroenterology 108:581–583

11. Days SP, Murphy P, Brown EA, Lemon SM (1992) Mutations within the 5' nontranslated region of hepatitis A virus RNA which enhance replication in BS-C-1 cells. J Virol 66:6533–6540

12. Schultz DE, Honda M, Whetter LE, McKnight KL, Lemon SM (1996) Mutations within the 5' nontranslated RNA of cell culture-adapted hepatitis A virus which enhance cap-independent translation in cultured African green monkey kidney cells. J Virol 70:1041–1049

Mutation Pattern of Hepatitis C Virus and Its Application to Therapy

Masashi Mizokami, Tatsunori Nakano, and Etsuro Orito

Introduction

Chronic hepatitis C is a common disease worldwide and is a major cause of chronic liver disease in many countries. However, the current standard therapy of chronic hepatitis C with interferon (IFN) is rather unsatisfactory [1-3]. Therefore, the search for additional therapies needs to be pursued. Molecular evolutionary analysis has been applied to numerous studies of hepatitis C virus (HCV) and has given many informative suggestions. However, it has not yielded helpful information for developing effective antiviral drugs against chronic HCV infection.

On the other hand, human immunodeficiency virus (HIV) infection has been one of the controllable diseases, owing to the development of combination therapy with a protease inhibitor, 3'-azido-2',3'-dideoxythymidine (AZT) and 2',3'-dideoxy-3'-thiacytidine (3TC) [4]. AZT is an analog of thymidine (T), and was reported to inhibit HIV replication to serve as a chain terminator of the HIV reverse transcriptase (RT) reaction instead of the true substrate [5]. AZT is more effective than other nucleoside analogs and is the most appropriate agent among nucleoside analogs for combination therapy against HIV infection [4,6,7]. However, the reason for the efficacy of AZT in preventing HIV replication remains to be determined. Moriyama et al. analyzed the nucleotide substitution patterns of genomes of HIV, and suggested that the high incidence of guanine (G) to adenine (A) substitution could be one of the reasons for the higher efficacy of AZT [8].

We analyzed nucleotide substitution patterns of HCV genomes using the same method adopted by Moriyama et al. and identified a nature of

Second Department of Medicine, Nagoya City University Medical School, 1 Mizuho-cho, Mizuho-ku, Nagoya 467-8601, Japan nucleotide substitution of HCV and furthermore, a unique substitution pattern of HCV during IFN therapy. It is expected that combination therapy using IFN and other potentially useful drugs will be as effective as combination therapy against HIV infection. We suggest new candidates of combination therapy with IFN against chronic hepatitis C, based on the results of nucleotide substitution patterns acquired from molecular evolutionary analysis of HCV genomes.

Materials and Methods

Patients

Five patients with chronic HCV infection were treated with IFN-α. They were seropositive for anti-HCV antibody and for HCV RNA by reverse transcription–polymerase chain reaction (RT-PCR). All patients received 6 million units (MU) of IFN intramuscularly for 2 weeks (six times a week), followed by 6 MU three times a week for an additional 22 weeks (468 MU in total). All the patients were followed up once a month for at least 6 months after the cessation of IFN therapy. Serum samples, taken just before the commencement and just after the cessation of IFN therapy, were used for the analysis for change of nucleotide substitution patterns in the E2 region of HCV during IFN therapy. All cases were infected with the genotype 1b strain of HCV.

RNA Extraction and Synthesis of cDNA

Two hundred μl of serum from each patient was employed for RNA extraction, and cDNA was generated from the extracted RNA with random priming using Moloney murine leukemia virus reverse transcriptase, at 37°C, for 60 min.

Detection and Genotyping of HCV RNA

Detection of HCV RNA was achieved by RT-PCR, using primers derived from the highly conserved 5' untranslated region [9]. HCV genotypes were determined by RT-PCR using genotype-specific primers derived from the core region, as described previously [10].

Sequencing of the HCV E2 Genomic Region

The HCV E2 genomic region was amplified under standard nested PCR conditions, using primers designed from the flank nucleotides 1105 to 1251 (nucleotide number according to the coding region of HCV-J; accession number: D90208) (5'-CAGYTRCTCCGGATCCCACAAGC-3' and 5'-ACGTCCGTCTCATTYKCVCCCCA-3'; and inner primers, 5'-TCTG-GATCCTATTCCATGGTGGGGAACTGG-3' (with a *Bam*HI site) and 5'-TCAGAATTCAGTCCTGTTGATRTGCCARCTGCC-3' (with an *Eco*RI site)). The PCR amplicons, which included hypervariable region 1 (HVR-1) [11], were digested by their respective restriction enzymes, and purified by gel electrophoresis, and were cloned into the pGEM-3zf(+) vector. Six clones each, from sera collected from each patient just before the commencement and just after the cessation of IFN treatment, were sequenced using the dideoxynucleotide chain termination method.

Analysis for Change of Nucleotide Substitution Patterns
in the HCV E2 Region During IFN Therapy

Six clones each, from sera collected from each patient just before the commencement and just after the cessation of IFN treatment, were aligned with an appropriate outer group sequence. To construct the phylogenetic trees, the number of nucleotide substitutions per site at all nucleotide positions was estimated by the 6-parameter method [12]. Based on these estimates, the phylogenetic trees were drawn using the neighbor-joining method [13], for each patient at two time points (Fig. 1). The roots of the trees were arbitrarily determined at the midpoint of the trees between six clones each and an outer group sequence. We chose a respective outer group sequence so that the genetic distances between all six clones of the same time point and the outer group sequence were almost equal. We could therefore assume that the node between each of the six clones and the outer group sequence was the ancestral nucleotide sequence of the six clones (represented by a solid circle in Fig. 1). We inferred the ancestral nucleotide sequences of these six clones site by site from the topology of the phylogenetic trees. Subsequently, we counted the numbers of the 12 kinds of nucleotide substitutions for each of the six clones, at all positions of codons. To analyze changes of the nucleotide substitution patterns during IFN therapy, the numbers counted from all

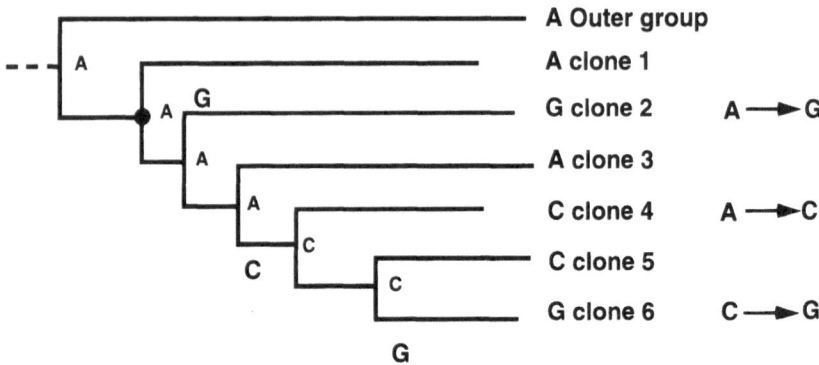

Fig. 1. The method for inferring the kind and number of 12 kinds of nucleotide substitution. Six clones each, from sera collected from each patient just before the commencement and just after the cessation of interferon (IFN) treatment, were aligned with an appropriate outer group sequence. To construct the phylogenetic trees, the number of nucleotide substitutions per site at all nucleotide positions was estimated by the 6-parameter method. Based on these estimates, the phylogenetic trees were drawn using the neighbor-joining method, for each patient at each time point. The roots of the trees were arbitrarily determined at the midpoint of the trees between six clones each and an outer group sequence. We chose a respective outer group sequence so that the genetic distances between all six clones of the same time point and the outer group sequence were almost equal. We could therefore assume that the node between each of the six clones and the outer group sequence was the ancestral nucleotide sequence of the six clones (represented by the *solid circle*). We decided the ancestral nucleotide sequences of these six clones site by site from the topology of the phylogenetic trees, and inferred the kind and number of 12 kinds of nucleotide substitution

five patients were added up at each time point, just before the commencement and just after the cessation of IFN treatment, respectively. Next, we computed the relative substitution frequencies for the 12 kinds of nucleotide substitution at each time point using the method by Gojobori et al. [14], correcting by the nucleotide composition of clones isolated at each time point. This value is more useful than the raw frequency of nucleotide change because it is unaffected by bias in the base composition in actual sequences. In this study, the nucleotide substitution pattern is shown as the set of 12 relative substitution frequencies. The relative substitution frequencies at the third position of codons were also analyzed in these five cases, based on the numbers of 12 kinds of substitution at the position.

Analysis of Nucleotide Substitution Patterns of HCV 1b Genomes
Inferred from the Phylogenies

To analyze nucleotide substitution patterns of HCV 1b, 22 HCV 1b strains
whose genome sequences encoding the full open reading frame were
registered in DNA databases (DDBJ, EMBL, and GenBank) were collected
from the HCV database (http://s2as02.genes.nig.ac.jp). These 22 HCV1b
sequences were aligned with a HCV 1a strain, HCV-1 (accession number:
M62321) in full coding region (nucleotide position: 1–9030). The phylogenetic tree was drawn using the same method described above. To determine the ancestral nucleotide sequence of these HCV 1b strains, we
constructed the phylogenetic tree of these 22 HCV 1b strains with HCV-
1 as an outer group sequence, and the root of the tree was arbitrarily
determined at the midpoint of the tree between 22 HCV 1b strains and
HCV-1. We considered that the branching point (node) between 22 HCV
1b strains and HCV-1 was the ancestral nucleotide sequence of these HCV
1b strains and continued to inferred ancestral nucleotide sequences of
these HCV 1b strains site by site from the topology of the phylogenetic
tree. We then counted the numbers of 12 kinds of nucleotide substitution,
respectively, at all positions of codons. Next, we computed the relative
substitution frequencies using the same method described above. The
relative substitution frequencies for 12 kinds of nucleotide substitution of
these 22 1b strains in the E2 region (nucleotide position: 1150–2427), at all
positions of codons were also analyzed using the method mentioned
above. The relative substitution frequencies at the third position of
codons were also analyzed in full coding or the E2 region, based on the
numbers of 12 kinds of substitution at the position.

Results

Nucleotide Substitution Patterns of 22 HCV 1b Strains Inferred
from the Phylogenies

These 22 HCV1b sequences were easily aligned with HCV-1 in the full
coding region, and the phylogenetic tree was constructed. From the
analysis of about 200 000 nucleotides of 22 HCV1b strains, we detected a
total of 8448 substitutions and computed the relative substitution frequencies in full coding region (Table 1). In the E2 region, these 22 HCV1b
sequences were easily aligned with HCV-1, and the phylogenetic tree was

Table 1. Substitution patterns at all positions of codons in each region of 22 HCV 1b clones

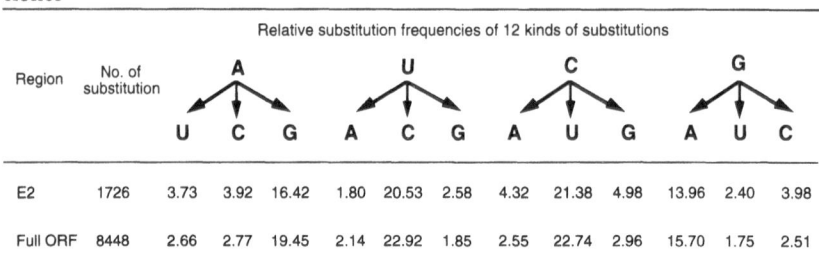

Region	No. of substitution	A→U	A→C	A→G	U→A	U→C	U→G	C→A	C→U	C→G	G→A	G→U	G→C
E2	1726	3.73	3.92	16.42	1.80	20.53	2.58	4.32	21.38	4.98	13.96	2.40	3.98
Full ORF	8448	2.66	2.77	19.45	2.14	22.92	1.85	2.55	22.74	2.96	15.70	1.75	2.51

constructed. From the tree and the alignment, we computed the relative substitution frequencies in the region.

Table 1 shows the relative substitution frequencies at all positions of codons in full coding region or the E2 region of 22 HCV1b strains. The frequencies of transitions, including adenine (A) to guanine (G), G to A, uridine (U) to cytosine (C), and C to U were high in full coding region and also in the E2 region. The same specific substitution patterns were also observed at the third position of codons (data not shown).

Biochemical and Virological Response to IFN Therapy of the Five Patients Analyzed by Nucleotide Substitution Patterns of HCV E2 Region

Figure 2 shows changes of the serum alanine aminotransferase (ALT) level (mean ± SD of five patients) in the five chronic hepatitis C patients treated with IFN-α. The serum ALT level was elevated just before the commencement of IFN therapy (154 ± 69 IU/l), and was normalized (<30 IU/l) by 2 months after the commencement of IFN therapy, followed thereafter by an increase in ALT level, in spite of continuation of IFN therapy. At the cessation of treatment, the ALT level was elevated (70 ± 46 IU/l). All cases showed a biochemical response to IFN but belonged to biochemical nonresponders for clinical criteria.

Changes of Nucleotide Substitution Patterns of HCV E2 Region During IFN Therapy

To determine the kind and number of nucleotide substitutions in each case at each time point, we constructed the phylogenetic trees of six

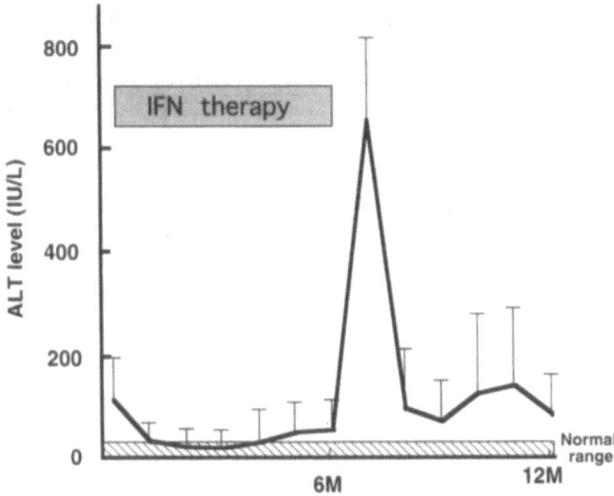

Fig. 2. Biochemical responses to IFN therapy of five patients analyzed by nucleotide substitution patterns of the E2 region of hepatitis C virus (HCV). Serum alanine aminotransferase (*ALT*) levels were followed up monthly from just before the commencement of IFN treatment to 6 months after the cessation of IFN. Serum ALT level of five patients was decreased during IFN therapy, followed thereafter by an increase again of ALT, in spite of continuation of IFN therapy. All cases exhibited biochemical responses to IFN

clones, with HCV-J as an outer group sequence, just before the commencement and just after the cessation of IFN treatment. We computed the relative substitution frequencies of the HCV E2 region in five cases at the two time points (Table 2). The frequency of U to C and C to U was high at each time point and did not change between the two time points. The same specific substitution pattern was also observed in the analysis of the third position of codons at each time point (data not shown).

Interestingly, the frequency of G to A at all positions increased significantly ($P < 0.05$) and that of A to G decreased significantly ($P < 0.05$) between before the commencement of and after the cessation of the IFN therapy (Table 2). Also, the frequency of G to A increased significantly ($P < 0.05$) and that of A to G decreased significantly ($P < 0.05$) between the two time points, in the analysis of the third position of codons (data not shown).

Table 2. Change of substitution patterns at all positions of codons before and after interferon (IFN) therapy in all cases

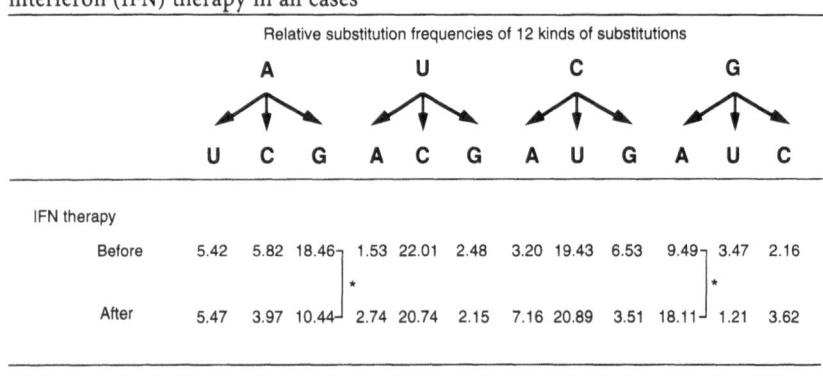

Relative substitution frequencies of 12 kinds of substitutions

	A			U			C			G		
IFN therapy	U	C	G	A	C	G	A	U	G	A	U	C
Before	5.42	5.82	18.46	1.53	22.01	2.48	3.20	19.43	6.53	9.49	3.47	2.16
After	5.47	3.97	10.44	2.74	20.74	2.15	7.16	20.89	3.51	18.11	1.21	3.62

*$P < 0.05$

Discussion

Generally, nucleotide substitution patterns are represented by spontaneous substitution mutations in genes free from any selective forces. In functional genes, nucleotide substitution patterns are affected by functional constraints at the amino acid level. However, the nucleotide substitution patterns at the third position of codons can reflect the spontaneous substitution mutation patterns in functional genes, since the nucleotide changes at the third position among such genes are mostly free from functional constraints. The relative substitution frequencies of transitions analyzed at all positions of codons were high in both full coding region and the E2 region of the 22 HCV1b strains. Moreover, the frequencies of transitions at the third position of codons were also high. It was suggested that transitional substitutions occurred easily in HCV genotype 1b. In the analysis of the HIV genomes, the nucleotide substitution patterns seem to result from the characteristics of the viral RT [8]. If that be so, then this specific substitution pattern may reflect the characteristics of RNA-dependent RNA polymerase of HCV, as HCV is replicated by RNA-dependent RNA polymerase. The frequencies of U to C and C to U were especially high in the E2 region of HCV isolated from sera of patients treated with IFN, and these substitutions were frequently observed in both clones isolated before and after IFN therapy. It is suggested that a high incidence of U to C and C to U substitutions is not affected by IFN, and is a characteristic of RNA-dependent RNA polymerase of HCV.

To investigate the influence of IFN on the substitution pattern of HCV, we chose the E2 region of HCV isolated from sera of patients treated with IFN. Since as many nucleotide substitutions as possible were needed to obtain a reliable relative substitution frequency, we analyzed this region at all positions of codons. This region includes a region encoding the envelope protein, since not only nucleotides at the third position but also even those at the first and second positions of codons in this region mutate more freely than those of other regions of HCV genome to escape the host immune system, we considered that the nucleotide substitutions at all positions of codons in this region reflected the spontaneous substitution pattern of the full coding region of HCV clones isolated before or after IFN. Actually, the substitution pattern at all positions was similar to the pattern at the third position, both before the commencement of and after the cessation of IFN therapy, and the pattern at all positions of the E2 region of HCV from patients was also similar to the pattern at all positions in the full coding region of 22 HCV1b strains derived from the DNA database (Tables 1 and 2). Moreover, a direct association of IFN therapy with the E2 region at the amino acid level has not been reported, although changes of quasispecies at this region related to IFN therapy have been reported [15]. Therefore, it is possible that the influence of IFN therapy on this region represents that on the full genome of HCV, although the mechanism by which IFN could exert influence on a change of the pattern is unknown.

We identified that the frequency of G to A substitution increased significantly and that of A to G decreased significantly in the analyzed region between before the commencement of and after the cessation of IFN therapy. Since we think that the nucleotide substitutions in this region reflect spontaneous substitution pattern of the entire coding region of HCV, it is supposed that a certain change in the character of RNA-dependent RNA polymerase of HCV has occurred during IFN therapy, as follows. In normal replication of HCV, complementary nucleotides corresponding to nucleotides in HCV RNA are incorporated into negative-strand RNA when HCV RNA is replicated to negative-strand RNA by RNA-dependent RNA polymerase of HCV (first step), and complementary nucleotides corresponding to the nucleotides in the negative strand RNA are incorporated into a new virus particle when a new HCV particle is propagated from the negative strand RNA by RNA-dependent RNA polymerase of HCV (second step). In G to A mutations, G in HCV RNA is replicated to incorrect U instead of correct C at the first step, and the U is

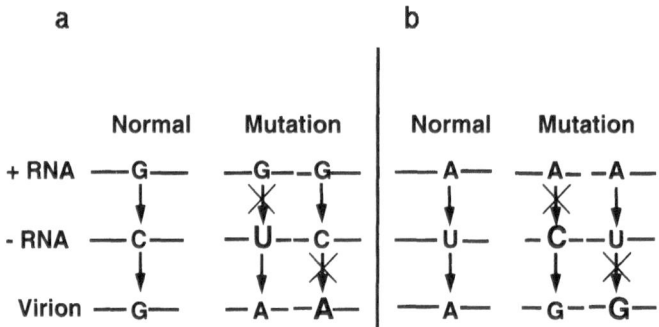

Fig. 3a,b. Mutation mechanism by HCV RNA-dependent RNA polymerase. **a** Normally, G in HCV RNA is replicated to complementary C in negative-strand RNA by RNA-dependent RNA polymerase of HCV (first step), and the C is replicated to complementary G in a new virus particle from the negative-strand RNA by RNA-dependent RNA polymerase of HCV (second step). In G to A mutations, G in HCV RNA are replicated to incorrect U instead of correct C at the first step, and the U is replicated to complementary A in a new virus particle at the second step; alternatively, G in HCV RNA is replicated to correct C at the first step, and the C is replicated to incorrect A instead of G in a new virus particle at the second step. Therefore, increase of G to A substitution during IFN therapy implies that incorrect U is more easily incorporated at the first step; alternatively, incorrect A is more easily incorporated at the second step during IFN therapy. **b** Decrease of A to G substitutions can be explained from the assumption that incorrect U or incorrect A is more easily incorporated at the first or second step, respectively, during IFN therapy. If U or A is more easily incorporated at the first and second step, respectively, A to U at the first step and U to A at the second step can easily occur, and can result in a decrease of A to G substitutions during IFN therapy

replicated to complementary A in a new virus particle at the second step; alternatively, G in HCV RNA is replicated to correct C at the first step, and the C is replicated to incorrect A instead of correct G in a new virus particle at the second step (Fig. 3a). Therefore, an increase of G to A substitutions during IFN therapy implies that incorrect U is more easily incorporated into negative-strand RNA at the first step; alternatively, incorrect A is more easily incorporated into a new virus particle at the second step during IFN therapy, by RNA-dependent RNA polymerase of HCV. A decrease of A to G substitutions can be explained from the assumption that incorrect U or incorrect A is more easily incorporated at the first or second step, respectively (Fig. 3b). Therefore, a decrease of A to G substitutions also supports the assumption that U or A is more easily incorporated at the first or second step, respectively, during IFN therapy. The assumption suggests possibilities of new combination therapies against HCV infection. Analogs or prodrugs of U or A might be candidates for combination therapy with IFN.

We obtained interesting results, which can be applied to clinical medicine, from molecular evolutionary analysis of the E2 region of HCV isolated from the sera of five patients. However, to determine whether our results are truly applicable to many other patients administered IFN, further studies are needed, with consideration of many factors such as genotype of HCV, quantification of HCV RNA, dose or term of IFN therapy, and biochemical or virological responses.

References

1. Carithers RLJ, Emerson SS (1997) Therapy of hepatitis C: meta-analysis of interferon alfa-2b trials. Hepatology 26(3 suppl 1):83S–88S
2. Farrell GC (1997) Therapy of hepatitis C: interferon alfa-n1 trials. Hepatology 26(3 suppl 1):96S–100S
3. Lee WM (1997) Therapy of hepatitis C: interferon alfa-2a trials. Hepatology 26(3 suppl 1):89S–95S
4. Carpenter CC, Fischl MA, Hammer SM, Hirsch MS, Jacobsen DM, Katzenstein DA, Montaner JS, Richman DD, Saag MS, Schooley RT, Thompson MA, Vella S, Yeni PG, Volberding PA (1997) Antiretroviral therapy for HIV infection in 1997. Updated recommendations of the International AIDS Society—USA panel. JAMA 277:1962–1969
5. De Clercq E (1995) Antiviral therapy for human immunodeficiency virus infections. Clin Microbiol Rev 8:200–239
6. Shirasaka T, Kavlick MF, Ueno T, Gao WY, Kojima E, Alcaide ML, Chokekijchai S, Roy BM, Arnold E, Yarchoan R, Mitsuya H (1995) Emergence of human immunodeficiency virus type 1 variants with resistance to multiple dideoxynucleosides in patients receiving therapy with dideoxynucleosides. Proc Natl Acad Sci USA 92:2398–2402
7. Shirasaka T, Chokekijchai S, Yamada A, Gosselin G, Imbach JL, Mitsuya H (1995) Comparative analysis of anti-human immunodeficiency virus type 1 activities of dideoxynucleoside analogs in resting and activated peripheral blood mononuclear cells. Antimicrob Agents Chemother 39:2555–2559
8. Moriyama EN, Ina Y, Ikeo K, Shimizu N, Gojobori T (1991) Mutation pattern of human immunodeficiency virus gene. J Mol Evol 32:360–363
9. Okamoto H, Okada S, Sugiyama Y, Tanaka T, Sugai Y, Akahane Y, Machida A, Mishiro S, Yoshizawa H, Miyakawa Y, Mayumi M (1990) Detection of hepatitis C virus RNA by a two-stage polymerase chain reaction with two pairs of primers deduced from the 5′-noncoding region. Jpn J Exp Med 60:215–222
10. Ohno O, Mizokami M, Wu RR, Saleh MG, Ohba K, Orito E, Mukaide M, Williams R, Lau JY (1997) New hepatitis C virus (HCV) genotyping system that allows for

identification of HCV genotypes 1a, 1b, 2a, 2b, 3a, 3b, 4, 5a, and 6a. J Clin Microbiol 35:201–207

11. Hijikata M, Kato N, Ootsuyama Y, Nakagawa M, Ohkoshi S, Shimotohno K (1991) Hypervariable regions in the putative glycoprotein of hepatitis C virus. Biochem Biophys Res Commun 175:220–228

12. Gojobori T, Ishii K, Nei M (1982) Estimation of average number of nucleotide substitutions when the rate of substitution varies with nucleotide. J Mol Evol 18:414–423

13. Saitou N, Nei M (1987) The neighbor-joining method: a new method for reconstructing phylogenetic trees. Mol Biol Evol 4:406–425

14. Gojobori T, Li WH, Graur D (1982) Patterns of nucleotide substitution in pseudogenes and functional genes. J Mol Evol 18:360–369

15. Enomoto N, Kurosaki M, Tanaka Y, Marumo F, Sato C (1994) Fluctuation of hepatitis C virus quasispecies in persistent infection and interferon treatment revealed by single-strand conformation polymorphism analysis. J Gen Virol 75(Pt 6):1361–1369

Randomized Controlled Trial of Lymphoblastoid Interferon-α for Chronic Hepatitis C; Early Disappearance of HCV RNA is Essential for Sustained Response

Shinichi Kakumu[1] and IFN Treatment Group of Affiliated Hospitals of the Third Department of Internal Medicine at Nagoya University School of Medicine

Introduction

Interferon (IFN) therapy has been shown to be efficacious in some patients with chronic hepatitis C [1–4]. In responders, normal alanine aminotransferase (ALT) levels and disappearance of hepatitis C virus (HCV) from serum continues for several years and probably permanently after IFN. Such a response is called sustained response, and has been thought to benefit the prognosis of the patients.

Three million units (MU) or 6 MU of IFNα is usually administered thrice weekly for 6 months. Increasing the dose of IFN has been reported to improve the rate of sustained response [5,6]. There are many retrospective studies on the efficacy of IFN focused on dose of the regimen and the predictive factors for sustained response for treatment of chronic hepatitis C. However, there are only a few prospective reports regarding these aspects. Thus, we conducted a randomized controlled trial to compare the efficacy of IFN between 6 MU and 9 MU. We also assessed the predictive factors for sustained response.

Patients and Methods

Patients

Eighty-four consecutive patients were enrolled in the study during April 1995 and July 1996. All patients had a histological diagnosis of

---

[1]First Department of Internal Medicine, Aichi Medical University, 21 Karimata Yazako, Nagakute-cho, Aichi-gun, Aichi 480-11, Japan

chronic hepatitis according to the international criteria [7]. The patients were positive for both serum anti-HCV antibody by second-generation enzyme-linked immunosorbent assay (Ortho Diagnostic System, Raritan, NJ, USA) and serum HCV RNA by Amplicor test (Nippon Roche, Tokyo, Japan). All of them had shown abnormal serum ALT levels on more than one occasion during the last 6 months before entering the study. The patients were negative for markers of vivid hepatitis B disease. Other causes of liver disease have been excluded in all patients. The study was approved by the local ethical committee and adhered to the ethical guidelines of the 1975 Declaration of Helsinki.

Treatment Schedule

The patients were randomly included in one of the two treatment groups using sealed envelopes. They were treated with lymphoblastoid IFNα (Sumitomo Pharmaceutical, Osaka, Japan) after giving informed consent; the doses were 6 MU for group A and 9 MU for group B. IFN was given intramuscularly daily for the first 2 weeks and then thrice weekly. IFN was continued for an additional 14 weeks, when HCV RNA became negative by Amplicor test at the second week of therapy. Otherwise the therapy was continued for 22 additional weeks. Sustained response was defined as ALT normalization and HCV RNA clearance maintained for more than 6 months after IFN therapy.

Genotyping and Quantitation of HCV RNA

Genotyping was done by HCV grouping assay, which detects genotype-specific antibodies in patients' sera (Immucheck-HCVGR Assay, International Reagents, Kobe, Japan) [8]. This assay discriminates between genotype 1 and 2 in Simmonds' classification [9]. Quantitation of HCV RNA was done by branched DNA assay (Quantiplex HCV RNA Assay, Chiron Corp., Emeryville, CA, USA) [10].

Statistical Evaluation

Univariate analysis was done by the chi-squared test and Student's *t*-test. Multivariate analysis was done by the logistic regression model.

Results and Discussion

Efficacy of Treatments

Two patients in group B withdrew from therapy because of adverse effects (depression for one and hallucination for the other). Two patients (1 in group A and 1 in group B) were lost before completing the follow-up period. Pretreatment biochemical and histological features of the 80 patients evaluated are shown in Table 1. There was no significant difference in each feature between the groups.

Twenty-two patients in group A (56.4%) and 28 in group B (68.3%) became negative for HCV RNA at the second week (not significant (NS)),

Table 1. Comparison of clinical, virological, and histological pretreatment features of the patients

	Group A	Group B	P-Value
No. of cases	39	41	NS
Age (years)[a]	51.0 ± 11.6	47.0 ± 11.8	NS
Male/female	24/15	30/11	NS
Presence of history of blood transfusion (+/−)	10/29	12/27	NS
ALT (IU/l)[a]	98.5 ± 64.1	105.5 ± 97.3	NS
Viral loads			
<1 Meq/ml	21	21	
≧1 Meq/ml	18	20	NS
Genotype 1	19	23	
2	18	17	NS
Undetermined	2	1	
Histology grading			
Minimal	2	0	
Mild	20	24	
Moderate	17	15	NS
Severe	0	2	
Staging			
1	1	1	
2	24	20	
3	14	20	NS

ALT, alanine aminotransferase; NS, not significant.
Statistical analysis was done by the chi- squared test and Student's t-test.
[a] Data expressed as mean ± SD.

who received IFN for an additional 14 weeks, and the rest of the patients received IFN for a further 22 weeks.

At the end of therapy, 26 patients is group A (66.7%) and 28 in group B (68.3%) had normal ALT levels (NS), and 27 patients in group A (69.2%) and 33 in group B (80.5%) became negative for HCV RNA (NS).

After IFN therapy, 17 patients in group A (43.6%) and 16 in group B (39.0%) sustained normal ALT levels for more than 6 months (NS), and 15 patients in group A (38.5%) and 16 in group B (39.0%) sustained negative results for HCV RNA (NS). The number of sustained responders who obtained both ALT normalization and HCV RNA clearance sustained for more than 6 months after IFN therapy was 14 in group A (35.9%) and 15 in group B (36.6%) (NS).

Predictive Factors for Sustained Response

Since there were no differences in the rate of sustained response between the two groups of patients, the predictive factors for sustained response were analyzed by combining the groups.

The following factors were evaluated: age, gender, presence of history of blood transfusion, pretreatment ALT levels, grading and staging of liver histology, viral loads, genotype, and negativity of HCV RNA at the second week of IFN therapy.

Univariate analysis showed that male gender, low viral loads (<1.0 Meq/ml), genotype 2, and negativity of HCV RNA at the second week of IFN were predictive for sustained response (Table 2). Twenty-eight of 29 sustained responders (96.6%) became negative for HCV RNA at the second week of therapy and the remaining patient became negative at the fourth week, while only 22 of 51 nonresponders (43.1%) became negative for HCV RNA at the second week ($P < 0.0001$).

Multivariate analysis demonstrated negativity of HCV RNA at the second week of IFN (odds ratio (OR), 50.0 and 95% confidence intervals (CI), 3.4–1000) and low viral loads (OR, 14.5 and 95% CI, 2.5–83.3) as the predictors for sustained response (Table 3).

Increasing the dosages of IFN has been reported to improve its efficacy in the treatment of chronic hepatitis C [5,6]. Chemello et al. reported a 12-month regimen starting with 6 MU of IFNα2a three times a week and then decreasing the dose was superior to the fixed dose of 3 MU three times a week for 12 months; the sustained response rate was 49% for the former and 31% for the latter [5]. Shiratori et al. reported that 9 MU of

Table 2. Univariate analysis for the predictors of sustained response

	Sustained responders	Nonresponders	P-Value
No. of cases	29	51	
Age (years)[a]	48.0 ± 13.3	52.0 ± 9.5	NS
Male/female	25/4	29/22	<0.05
Presence of history of blood transfusion (+/−)	5/24	17/34	NS
ALT (IU/l)[a]	98.5 ± 54.7	103.5 ± 87.7	NS
Viral loads			
<1 Meq/ml	26	16	
≧1 Meq/ml	3	35	<0.001
Genotype 1	10	32	
2	17	18	<0.001
Undetermined	2	1	
Histology grading			
Minimal	0	2	
Mild	18	26	
Moderate	10	22	NS
Severe	1	1	
Staging			
1	1	1	
2	16	28	
3	12	22	NS
HCV RNA at the second week of IFN (+/−)	1/28	29/32	<0.0001

HCV, hepatitis C virus; IFN, interferon; NS, not significant.
Statistical analysis was done by the chi- squared test and Student's t-test.
[a] Data expressed as mean ± SD.

Table 3. Multivariate analysis for predictors of sustained response

Factor	Odds ratio	95% Confidence interval
Negative HCV RNA at second week	50.0	3.4–1000
Viral load <1 Meq/ml	14.5	2.5–83.3
Gender (male)	4.8	0.8–28.4

lymphoblastoid IFNα administered three times a week for 6 months produced a high virus eradication rate compared with that of 6 MU (36% vs 25%, $P < 0.05$) at 12 months after completion of treatment [6]. However, there have been few randomized trials to compare the efficacy of an increased dose with that of the usual dose for 6 months. Our randomized

controlled trial indicated that there was no difference in sustained response rate between 6 MU and 9 MU of lymphoblastoid IFNα for 16–24
weeks. Therefore, it is still unresolved whether we treat the patients with
6 MU or 9 MU of IFNα.

Univariate analysis showed that male gender, low viral loads
(<1.0 Meq/ml), genotype 2, and HCV RNA negativity at the second week
of IFN were predictive for sustained response. Multivariate analysis demonstrated that negativity of HCV RNA at the second week of IFN and low
viral loads were significant predictors for sustained response. Similar
prognostic parameters have been reported: low viral loads, mild fibrosis,
genotype other than genotype 1, and early disappearance of HCV RNA by
IFN [11–16]. The present study confirmed these previous findings including our retrospective reports.

All the sustained responders but one became negative for HCV RNA by
Amplicor test at the second week of therapy, and even the one exception
became negative at the fourth week, while more than half to the
nonresponders were positive at the second week. Thus the earlier disappearance of HCV RNA at the second week or at least the fourth week is an
essential condition for sustained response. When we consider the sustained response as the only goal of IFN therapy for chronic hepatitis C, it
is possible to identify more than half of the patients who would become
nonresponders at the second or at least the fourth week, and to stop
further therapy. This approach would save the enormous expense of IFN
therapy for nonresponders.

However, it has been suggested that the transient normalization of ALT
levels may benefit the clinical course of the patients [17]. Actually, 72.5%
(37/51) of nonresponders in the present study normalized their ALT
levels during treatment. In addition, some nonresponders sustain normal
ALT levels for a considerably long time despite the presence of HCV RNA
after IFN therapy [18,19]. Whether temporary or long-lasting normalization of ALT levels would benefit patients is yet to be determined. To
establish an efficient strategy of IFN therapy for chronic hepatitis C, we
need to know whether the nonresponders would benefit from IFN
therapy.

Summary

To assess the efficacy and predictive factors of two different dosages of
lymphoblastoid IFNα, a randomized controlled trial was conducted.

Eighty-four patients with chronic hepatitis C were enrolled into the trial and 80 patients were evaluated. Thirty-nine patients were treated with 6 MU (group A) and 41 patients with 9 MU (group B) daily for the first 2 weeks, and then thrice weekly. The therapy was continued for an additional 14 weeks, when HCV RNA became negative by Amplicor test at the second week of therapy. Otherwise it was continued for an additional 22 weeks. Fourteen patients in group A (35.9%) and 15 in group B (36.6%) attained sustained response. Multivariate analysis demonstrated negativity of HCV RNA at the second week of IFN (OR, 50.0) and low viral loads (OR, 14.5) as the predictors for sustained response. Twenty-eight of 29 sustained responders became negative for HCV RNA at the second week of therapy, while only 22 of 51 nonresponders became negative ($P < 0.0001$). The results of the present trial indicated that there was no difference in sustained response rate between 6 MU and 9 MU doses, and that almost all the sustained responders became negative for HCV RNA at the second week of therapy. Thus the earlier disappearance of HCV RNA at the second week or at least the fourth week is an essential condition for sustained response.

References

1. Davis GL, Balart LA, Schiff ER, et al (1989) Treatment of chronic hepatitis C with recombinant interferon alpha. A multicenter randomized, controlled trial. N Engl J Med 321:1501–1506
2. Di Bisceglie AM, Martin P, Kassianides C, et al (1989) Recombinant interferon alpha therapy for chronic hepatitis C. A randomized, double-blind, placebo-controlled trial. N Engl J Med 321:1506–1510
3. Marcellin P, Boyer N, Giostra E, et al (1991) Recombinant human alpha-interferon in patients with chronic non-A, non-B hepatitis: a multicenter randomized controlled trial from France. Hepatology 13:393–397
4. Pagliaro L, Craxi A, Cammaa C, et al (1994) Interferon-alpha for chronic hepatitis C: an analysis of pretreatment clinical predictors of response. Hepatology 19:820–828
5. Chemello L, Bonetti P, Cavalletto L, et al (1995) Randomized trial comparing three different regimens of alpha-2a-interferon in chronic hepatitis C. Hepatology 22:700–706
6. Shiratori Y, Kato N, Yokosuka O, et al (1997) Predictors of the efficacy of interferon therapy in chronic hepatitis C virus infection. Gastroenterology 113:558–566
7. Desmet VJ, Gerber M, Hoofnagle JH, et al (1994) Classification of chronic hepatitis: diagnosis, grading and staging. Hepatology 19:1513–1520

8. Tanaka T, Tsukiyama-Kohara K, Yamaguchi K, et al (1994) Significance of specific antibody assay for genotyping of hepatitis C virus. Hepatology 19:1347–1353
9. Simmonds P, McOmish F, Yap PL, et al (1993) Sequence variability in the 5' noncoding region of hepatitis C virus: identification of a new virus type and restrictions on sequence diversity. J Gen Virol 74:661–668
10. Urdea MS, Horn T, Fultz TJ, et al (1991) Branched DNA amplification multimers for the sensitive, direct detection of human hepatitis viruses. Nucleic Acids Symp Ser 24:197–200
11. Lau JYN, Davis GL, Kniffen J, et al (1993) Significance of serum hepatitis C virus RNA levels in chronic hepatitis C. Lancet 341:1501–1504
12. Yoshioka K, Higashi Y, Yamada M, et al (1995) Predictive factors in the response to interferon therapy in chronic hepatitis C. Liver 15:57–62
13. Yoshioka K, Kakumu S, Wakita T, et al (1992) Detection of hepatitis C virus by polymerase chain reaction and response to interferon-alpha therapy: relationship to genotypes of hepatitis C virus. Hepatology 16:293–299
14. Hino K, Okuda M, Konishi T, et al (1995) Serial assay of hepatitis C virus RNA in serum for predicting response to interferon-alpha therapy. Dig Dis Sci 40:14–20
15. Orito E, Mizokami M, Suzuki K, et al (1995) Loss of serum HCV RNA at week 4 of interferon-alpha therapy is associated with more favorable long-term response in patients with chronic hepatitis C. J Med Virol 46:109–115
16. Kakumu S, Aiyama T, Okumura A, et al (1997) Earlier loss of hepatitis C virus RNA in interferon therapy can predict a long-term response in chronic hepatitis C. J Gastroenterol Hepatol 12:468–472
17. Sharara AI, Hunt CM, Hamilton JD (1996) Hepatitis C. Ann Intern Med 125:658–668
18. Kakumu S, Yoshioka K, Tanaka K, et al (1993) Long-term carrier state of hepatitis C virus with normal aminotransferase after interferon treatment in patients with chronic hepatitis C. J Med Virol 41:65–70
19. Lau JY, Mizokami M, Ohno T, et al (1993) Discrepancy between biochemical and virological responses to interferon-alpha in chronic hepatitis C. Lancet 342:1208–1209

Use of Interferon-α for Prevention of Hepatocellular Carcinoma in Patients with Chronic Active Hepatitis C with Cirrhosis

S. Nishiguchi, S. Nakatani, A. Tamori, T. Takeda, S. Shiomi, S. Seki, and T. Kuroki

Introduction

Hepatitis C virus (HCV) is a more important factor associated with hepatocellular carcinoma than hepatitis B virus (HBV) in Japan and certain Western countries [1–3]. Some patients who contracted chronic non-A, non-B hepatitis after blood transfusion and hepatocellular carcinoma many years later have been studied in detail [4–6]. These studies proved that patients with chronic HCV infection often develop hepatocellular carcinoma [7]. The cumulative incidence of hepatocellular carcinoma in patients who had blood transfusions and were negative for hepatitis B surface antigen (HBsAg) was 53% (13/26) during 6 years of observation [8]. All of these patients had HCV antibodies. The mechanism by which hepatocellular carcinoma develops in the presence of HCV is unknown.

After Hoofnagle et al. [9] reported the efficacy of interferon (IFN) in non-A, non-B chronic active hepatitis (CAH), several randomized controlled trials have shown that IFN therapy leads to a rapid decrease in serum alanine aminotransferase (ALT) activity and to a disappearance of serum HCV RNA in about one-third of patients with chronic hepatitis C [10,11]. Patients who respond to IFN therapy with long-term remission of disease and the sustained loss of HCV RNA are not likely to develop cirrhosis of the liver or hepatocellular carcinoma. Most hepatocellular carcinoma with underlying HCV is detected at the cirrhotic stage of hepatitis. In Japan, the reported interval from blood transfusion to diagnosis

Third Department of Internal Medicine, Osaka City University Medical School, 1-5-7 Asahi-machi, Abeno-ku, Osaka 545-8586, Japan
Supported in part by a grant from the Ministry of Welfare, Japan

of cirrhosis has been 20 to 25 years; the interval between blood transfusion and diagnosis of hepatocellular carcinoma has been about 30 years
[12]. We planned this trial of prevention of carcinogenesis by IFN in
cirrhotic patients with HCV infection because of their high risk of
hepatocellular carcinoma.

Subjects and Methods

Patients

During the 10 years from January 1988 to December 1997, we studied 90
patients with CAH and cirrhosis of the liver diagnosed clinically. Histological findings were assessed by the histological activity index (HAI) of
Knodell et al. [13]. Patients fulfilled all of the following criteria: (1) abnormal serum ALT levels for at least 1 year before entry; (2) absence of
HBsAg and other explanations (such as habitual drinking or autoimmune
liver disease) of chronic liver disease except for HCV; (3) compensated
cirrhosis of grade A by the Child-Pugh score [14] (total bilirubin <2 mg/
dl, serum albumin >2.8 g/dl, prothrombin time 1–4 s, and no signs of
ascites or hepatic encephalopathy); (4) absence of severe thrombocytopenia (defined as <50 000/mm^3); (5) absence of antibodies to human
immunodeficency virus; (6) presence of HCV RNA (this criterion was
applied retrospectively for patients selected in 1988 and 1989, and serum
was tested for HCV antibodies as well); (7) absence of hepatocellular
carcinoma or a suspicious-looking space-occupying region found by
ultrasonography and computerized tomography. For patients who
entered in 1988 and 1989, blood was sampled and serum was obtained
and kept frozen; HCV antibodies and HCV RNA were assayed later.
All patients had HCV antibodies and HCV RNA. Starting in 1990,
we assayed HCV antibodies and HCV RNA at the time of entry.
All patients were enrolled between January 1988 and June 1992. After
written informed consent was obtained, each patient was randomly
assigned to treatment with IFN-α or symptomatic treatment [15].
All procedures during the trial were in accordance with the Helsinki
Declaration of 1975 as revised in 1983, and were approved by the
appropriate committee at Osaka City University Medical School. IFN
almost invariably causes a high fever. In this study, it was injected intramuscularly 36–72 times. If the trial were to be a double-blind one, a
placebo that caused fever would have to be injected many times. Such a

placebo was not acceptable to us; it was rejected for reasons described by Hill [16].

Treatment

Ninety patients were allocated by reference to a table of random numbers to a group given IFN or a control group. The 45 patients in the IFN group received 6 MIU of IFN-α (human lymphoblastoid interferon; Sumiferon, Sumitomo Pharmaceuticals, Osaka, Japan) intramuscularly three times a week for 12 to 24 weeks. Ten of these patients received the lower daily dose (3 MIU) because of side effects, especially severe thrombocytopenia. After the first treatment ended, 6 patients chose to receive IFN treatment again, and one of these patients received the same treatment three times. The 45 control patients received symptomatic therapy to treat ascites or the like, and dietary advice, but did not receive any antiviral therapy or immunomodulatory therapy, such as with corticosteroids.

Evaluation of Therapeutic Response

All patients were then seen every 3 months for at least 2 years. At each visit, the patients reported the clinical manifestations of their disease. Blood and urine samples were obtained for blood counts, biochemical tests, and virologic studies. All patients were prospectively monitored by measurement of serum levels of α-fetoprotein (AFP) and by ultrasonographic scanning every 3 months. Ultrasonography was done by specialists not aware of the treatment being given, with a convex-array real-time scanner (3.5 MHz, model SSD 650, Aloka, Tokyo, Japan; EUB 340 and 415, Hitachi Medical, Tokyo, Japan; and model SSA 90A, Toshiba Systems, Tokyo, Japan). Selective hepatic angiography was performed when hepatocellular carcinoma was suspected. The diagnosis of hepatocellular carcinoma was checked by histological inspection of a specimen obtained by ultrasound-guided biopsy when indicated.

Serum ALT, serum albumin, serum γ-globulin, and total bilirubin levels were assayed with an Autoanalyzer 7450 (Hitachi, Tokyo, Japan). Peripheral blood cells were counted by a Sysmex NE-8000 apparatus (Toa Medical Electronics, Kobe, Japan) and the serum AFP was measured with a Pamia-100 apparatus (Toa). Anti-HCV antibodies were measured with a first- or second-generation enzyme-linked immunosorbent assay

(Ortho Diagnostics, Tokyo, Japan). Serum HCV RNA was detected by reverse transcription and a nested polymerase chain reaction with primers derived from the highly conserved 5'-untranslated region of the viral genome, as described previously [17]. Each test was done by two investigators and was checked for agreement by a third investigator. Only reproducible results obtained in at least two independent experiments were considered in this study. For the purpose of this trial, we defined a response as the disappearance of HCV RNA from the serum. We considered therapy to be effective if HCV RNA disappeared by the end of therapy and could not be detected during follow-up. HCV genotypes were identified by the method of Okamoto et al. [18].

Statistical Methods

Statistical analysis was done with SAS software (SAS Institute, Cary, NC, USA). Fisher's exact test was used to evaluate the significance of the differences in the ratios of sex and HCV genotypes in the groups. The distribution of the data was checked by normal probability plots. Student's t-test was used to analyze the differences in age, platelet counts, serum albumin concentrations, and HAI, and the Wilcoxon rank-sum test was used to assess the differences in the serum ALT level and AFP level. The cumulative incidence of hepatocellular carcinoma was plotted by the Kaplan-Meier method, and the statistical significance of differences in this incidence was found by the Gehan modification of the generalized Wilcoxon signed rank test. Cox's regression model using proportional hazards was used for multivariate analysis. All P-values are two-tailed. A P-value below 0.05 was considered to indicate statistical significance.

Results

Characteristics of the Patients

The characteristics of the 90 patients who were not excluded and who gave consent to participate were evaluated immediately after entry (Table 1). The patients in the IFN and control groups were similar with respect to mean age, sex ratio, levels of serum albumin, ALT, and AFP, platelet count, numbers with different HCV genotypes, and total HAI as defined by Knodell et al. [19].

Table 1. Baseline characteristics of control patients and patients given interferon (IFN)-α

Characteristic	Control group	IFN group	P-Value
Age (years)[a]	57.3 ± 6.9	54.7 ± 5.8	0.065
Sex (M/F)	23/22	28/170.395	
Albumin (g/dl)[a]	3.7 ± 0.4	3.7 ± 0.3	0.686
ALT	100 (67–125)	117 (95–134)	0.132
AFP	6 (5–23)	12 (7–39)	0.095
Platelets (10^{-4}/mm^3)[a]	9.7 ± 4.5	10.1 ± 4.3	0.840
HCV genotypes			
I	0	1	0.685
II	33	35	
II	8	6	
IV	4	3	
V	0	0	
HAI	11.8 ± 2.7	11.7 ± 2.7	0.829

The statistical significance of differences was calculated by Student's *t*-test, Wilcoxon rank-sum test, or Fisher's exact test. No statistically significant differences were found between the group given IFN and the control group. Alanine aminotransferase (ALT) and α-fetoprotein (AFP) levels are expressed as medians (with 25th and 75th percentiles). The histological activity index (HAI) was assessed by the method of Knodell et al. [13].
HCV, hepatitis C virus.
[a] Means ± SD are given.

Response to IFN-α

At the start of the trial, all patients in the two groups had HCV RNA in their serum. At the end of the therapy, HCV RNA was not detected in 16 of the 45 patients who had received IFN-α. However, at the end of the follow-up period, only 7 patients remained negative for HCV RNA. Of these 7 patients, all had decreased serum ALT activity (<40 IU), and the level has remained normal to date. HCV RNA disappeared in none of the control patients ($P = 0.018$), and the ALT activity did not become normal in any of these patients. Late in follow-up, the patients given IFN had a mean ALT level lower than their baseline level and lower than in the control group (Fig. 1). The AFP level increased gradually in the control group 4 years after entry and was higher than in the group given IFN (both $P < 0.05$; data not shown). The group given IFN had a higher serum albumin level after treatment than before treatment or than that of the control group (both $P < 0.01$; Fig. 2).

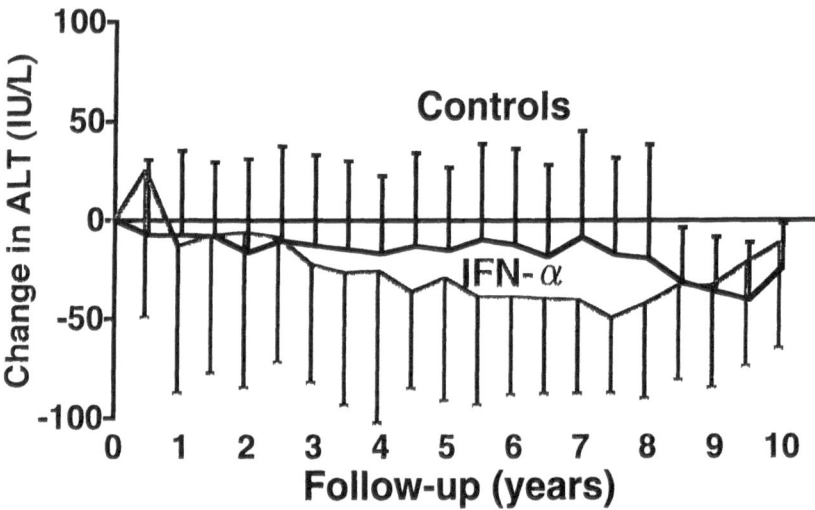

Fig. 1. Serum alanine aminotransferase (*ALT*) levels in group given interferon-α (*IFN*-α) and control group during follow-up. The *dark line* shows the medians of the group given IFN-α and the *black line* shows medians for the control group. *Vertical bars* indicate the 25th and 75th percentiles

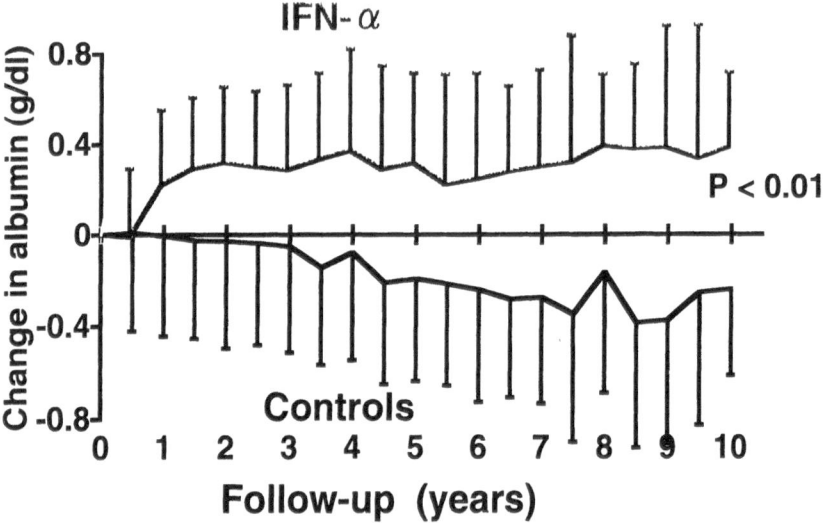

Fig. 2. Serum albumin levels in group given IFN and control group during follow-up. The *dark line* shows the medians of the group given *IFN*-α and the *black line* shows medians for the control group. *Vertical bars* indicate SD

Development of Hepatocellular Carcinoma

The mean follow-up period for both groups was more than 7 years. Of the 45 patients given IFN, 9 were found to have hepatocellular carcinoma. In these patients, treatment had been judged to be ineffective because HCV RNA did not disappear and serum ALT did not decrease after the start of therapy. Twenty-nine of the controls were found to have hepatocellular carcinoma during follow-up. IFN significantly decreased the cumulated incidence of hepatocellular carcinoma (data not shown). The conditional risk ratio was calculated with 7 variables (age, sex, serum albumin level, ALT level, AFP level, platelet count, and type of treatment) by multivariate analysis of Cox's regression model using proportional hazards. The conditional risk ratio of the group given IFN vs the control group was 0.196 ($P = 0.001$).

Discussion

The main aim of this study is to elucidate whether interferon reduces the incidence of hepatocellular carcinoma. After we published the data of this study [19], several studies were reported concerning the incidence of hepatocellular carcinoma in relation to interferon. Mazella et al. [20] reported that the incidence and the risk of developing hepatocellular carcinoma was reduced by IFN-α. However, Fattovich et al. [21] reported that their analysis did not detect any significant benefit of IFN-α on estimated probability of the occurrence of hepatocellular carcinoma. These two studies are not randomized prospective studies, therefore the difference in the backgrounds between the control group and the IFN-treated group can change the final results. The relatively low number of events in these studies may also give the explanation for the different results.

In patients with chronic infection by HCV, especially those with CAH with cirrhosis, the virus has been directly linked to the development of hepatocellular carcinoma [7]. The mechanism of malignant transformation is not known, because this is an RNA virus without reverse transcriptase activity, so the integration in host DNA that usually occurs in subjects infected with HBV is unlikely with HCV. There are no reports that a gene related to HCV causes transactivation of a cellular gene, as does an HBX gene [22]. The accumulation of genetic alternations was first described by Vogelstein et al. [23] as stepwise carcinogenesis. The frequency of activation of protooncogenes and inactivation of suppressor genes probably increase as hepatocytes replicate. Such replication is more vigorous when cells are continuously damaged and therefore replaced by regeneration, as in CAH with or without cirrhosis during chronic infection by HCV [24]. In other words, the rate of cell division affects the possibility of carcinogenesis, and if chronic infection by HCV is cured, carcinogenesis in the liver might be prevented. In patients for whom IFN is effective (HCV RNA disappears, and serum ALT level enters and remains in the normal range), carcinogenesis is unlikely, because the rate of cell division decreased in such patients. If our patients for whom IFN was effective even had a small hepatocellular carcinoma or precancerous lesion, such as adenomatous hyperplasia, which could not detected by ultrasonography before treatment, curing of the chronic infection might delay growth of the cancer to detectable size. In this trial, 7 patients with CAH with cirrhosis for whom treatment with IFN was effective have not developed hepatocellular carcinoma 5, 5, 6, 6, 8, 8, and 9 years, respectively, after treatment. However, in most patients, HCV RNA disappeared transiently or did not disappear with IFN treatment, and they could have developed hepatocellular carcinoma at any time. Even in the patients for whom treatment was ineffective, as judged by HCV RNA levels, the mean serum ALT and AFP levels decreased, and the serum albumin level increased significantly after IFN treatment. These results show that the inflammation of Glisson's capsule and necrosis of the hepatocytes became milder with treatment, and that movement of hepatocytes through the cell cycle slowed. Therefore, the incidence of accumulated genetic abnormalities occurring during cell division might be lower in the patients for whom IFN was ineffective than if the patients had not been given IFN.

Summary

The role of IFN in reducing the incidence of hepatocellular carcinoma is still controversial. In a prospective randomized controlled trial, the effects of IFN on carcinogenesis were compared with those of symptomatic treatment including dietary advice in 90 patients with compensated CAH C with cirrhosis. Patients were randomly allocated to a group given 6 MU of IFN-α three times weekly for 12 to 24 weeks or to a control group given symptomatic treatment. Patients were monitored for 2 to 9 years for hepatocellular carcinoma by ultrasonography and assays of AFP. Late in follow-up, mean ALT activity in patients given IFN tended to be lower than in the controls. The serum albumin level in the group given IFN was higher than in the controls (both $P < 0.001$). Hepatitis C viral RNA disappeared and ALT remained normal in 7 of the 45 patients given IFN, and in none of the 45 controls ($P = 0.001$). The incidence of hepatocellular carcinoma was 9 patients given IFN and 29 controls ($P = 0.001$ by Kaplan-Meier analysis). The conditional risk ratio of IFN vs controls was 0.196 ($P = 0.0001$ by Cox's regression model using proportional hazards). IFN-α improved liver function in CAH C with cirrhosis and helped to prevent hepatocellular carcinoma.

Acknowledgments. The authors thank Ms. H. Fujimoto and Ms. E. Maekawa for technical assistance, and K. Nukui for statistical analysis.

References

1. Bruix J, Barrera JM, Calvet X, et al (1989) Prevalence of antibodies to hepatitis C virus in Spanish patients with hepatocellular carcinoma and hepatic cirrhosis. Lancet ii:1004–1006
2. Colombo M, Kuo G, Choo QL, et al (1989) Prevalence of antibodies to hepatitis C virus in Italian patients with hepatocellular carcinoma. Lancet ii:1006–1008
3. Nishioka K, Watanabe J, Furuta S, et al (1991) A high prevalence of antibody to the hepatitis C virus in patients with hepatocellular carcinoma in Japan. Cancer 67:429–433
4. Resnick RH, Stone K, Antonioli D (1983) Primary hepatocellular carcinoma following non-A, non-B posttransfusion hepatitis. Dig Dis Sci 28:908–911
5. Kiyosawa K, Akahane Y, Nagata A, Furuta S (1984) Hepatocellular carcinoma after non-A, non-B posttransfusion hepatitis. Am J Gastroenterol 79:777–781
6. Gilliam JH II, Geisinger KR, Richter JE (1984) Primary hepatocellular carcinoma after chronic non-A, non-B post-transfusion hepatitis. Ann Intern Med 101:794–795
7. Tremolada F, Benvegnu L, Casarin C, Pontisso P, Tagger A Alberti A (1990) Antibody to hepatitis C virus in hepatocellular carcinoma. Lancet 335:300–301
8. Oka H, Kurioka N, Kim K, et al (1990) Prospective study of early detection of hepatocellular carcinoma in patients with cirrhosis. Hepatology 12:680–687
9. Hoofnagle JH, Mullen KD, Jones DB, et al (1986) Treatment of chronic non-A, non-B hepatitis with recombinant human alpha interferon: a preliminary report. N Engl J Med 315:1575–1578
10. Di Bisceglie AM, Martin P, Kassianides C, et al (1989) Recombinant interferon alpha therapy for chronic hepatitis C: a randomized, double-blind placebo-controlled trial. N Engl J Med 321:1506–1510
11. Shindo M, Di Bisceglie AM, Hoofnagle JH (1992) Long-term follow-up of patients with chronic hepatitis C treated with α-interferon. Hepatology 15:1013–1016

12. Kiyosawa K, Sodeyama T, Tanaka E, et al (1990) Interrelationship of blood transfusion, non-A, non-B hepatitis and hepatocellular carcinoma: analysis by detection of antibody to hepatitis C virus. Hepatology 12:671–675
13. Knodell RG, Ishak KG, Black WC, et al (1981) Formulation and application of a numerical scoring system for assessing histological activity in asymptomatic chronic active hepatitis. Hepatology 1:431–435
14. Pugh RNH, Murray-Lyon IM, Dawson JL, et al (1973) Transection of the oesophagus for bleeding oesophageal varices. Br J Surg 60:646–649
15. Sherlock S, Dooley J (1997) Diseases of the liver and biliary system, 9th edn. Blackwell, Oxford, p 367
16. Hill AB (1963) Medical ethics and controlled trials. Br Med J i:1043–1049
17. Nishiguchi S, Kuroki T, Ueda T, et al (1992) Detection of hepatitis C virus antibody in the absence of viral RNA in patients with autoimmune hepatitis. Ann Intern Med 116:21–25
18. Okamoto H, Tokita H, Sakamoto M, et al (1993) Characterization of the genomic sequence of type V (or 3a) hepatic C virus isolates and PCR primers for specific detection. J Gen Virol 74:2835–2890
19. Nishiguchi S, Kuroki T, Nakatani S, et al (1995) Randomised trial of effects of interferon-α on incidence of hepatocellular carcinoma in chronic active hepatitis C with cirrhosis. Lancet 346:1051–1056
20. Mazzella G, Accogli E, Sottili S, et al (1996) Alpha interferon treatment may prevent hepatocellular carcinoma in HCV-related liver cirrhosis. J Hepatol 24:141–147
21. Fattovich G, Giustina G, Degos F, et al (1997) Effectiveness of interferon alpha on incidence of hepatocellular carcinoma and decompensation in cirrhosis type C. J Hepatol 27:201–205
22. Chisari FV, Klopchin K, Moriyama T, et al (1989) Molecular pathogenesis of hepatocellular carcinoma in hepatitis B virus transgenic mice. Cell 59:1145–1156
23. Vogelstein B, Fearon ER, Hamilton SR, et al (1988) Genetic alterations during colorectal-tumor development. N Engl J Med 319:525–532
24. Okuda K (1992) Hepatocellular carcinoma: recent progress. Hepatology 15:948–963

Risk Factors for Hepatocellular Carcinoma Among Chronic Hepatitis C Patients Treated with Interferon

AKINORI KASAHARA[1,2], NORIO HAYASHI[2], SHINICHI KAKUMU[3], KENDO KIYOSAWA[4], KIWAMU OKITA[5], and the OSAKA LIVER DISEASE STUDY GROUP

Introduction

In Japan, the incidence of hepatocellular carcinoma (HCC) has been increasing over the last 30 years, and epidemiological surveys have shown that as a causative agent, hepatitis C virus (HCV) is more common than hepatitis B virus (HBV). Chronic hepatitis C has been demonstrated to evolve to cirrhosis and HCC [1–3]. The HCC occurrence rate in cirrhotic patients with anti-HCV has been reported to increase steadily with a yearly incidence of 1.4%–7% [4–6]. Thus, a majority of cases with chronic HCV infection progress slowly to liver cirrhosis and HCC.

More than 200 000 Japanese patients with chronic hepatitis C have been treated with interferon. Many investigators have reported this therapy to be effective for decreasing serum alanine aminotransferase (ALT) [7,8], reducing and eliminating HCV RNA levels [9,10], and improving liver histology [11,12] in patients with chronic hepatitis C. However, there have been no studies on the relationship between the response to interferon therapy and the development of HCC after it. Therefore, we decided to evaluate the influence of interferon therapy on the development of HCC by exploring the risk factors for liver carcinogenesis and examining the incidence of HCC in chronic hepatitis C patients treated with interferon.

---

[1] Department of General Medicine, Osaka University Hospital, 2-15 Yamada-oka, Suita, Osaka 565-0871, Japan
[2] First-Department of Medicine, Osaka University School of Medicine, 2-2 Yamada-oka, Suita, Osaka 565-0871, Japan
[3] First-Department of Medicine, Aichi Medical School, Yazako, Ohaza, Nagakute-cho, Aichi 480-11, Japan
[4] Second-Department of Medicine, Shinshu University School of Medicine, 3-1-1 Asahi, Matsumoto, Nagano 390-0802, Japan
[5] First-Department of Medicine, Yamaguchi University School of Medicine, 1144 Kogushi, Ooaza, Ube, Yamaguchi 755-0067, Japan

Patients and Methods

Patient Studies

From June 1989 to September 1995, a total of 1142 patients, who had had elevated ALT (at least double the upper limit of the normal range for at least 6 months) and who had been histologically proven to have chronic hepatitis with or without Child grade A liver cirrhosis, were treated with interferon in six trials using defferent treatment schedules [9-11,13-15]. Patients with positive hepatitis B surface antigen, or other forms of liver disease (such as alcoholic liver disease and autoimmune liver disease) were excluded from the interferon treatment trials. Also excluded from the treatment trials were patients with ultrasonic coarse-nodular cirrhosis before the start of interferon therapy and those with a history of hepatic encephalopathy, bleeding esophageal varices, or ascites. The case was excluded from this study if the total amount of interferon was less than 200 million units (MU), because of the possibility of insufficient interferon treatment (39 cases). Also, patients developing HCC within 1 year after the completion of interferon therapy were not included, so as to exclude as many cases having microscopic HCC prior to interferon therapy as was possible (nine cases, all of whom were nonresponders). Patients with less than 12 months of follow-up using ultrasonography for miscellaneous reasons were also excluded (72 cases). After these procedures, 1022 patients were left and followed up in this study, none of whom were positive for HIV antibody.

For the first interferon treatment regimen, one group of 159 patients was randomly assigned to receive either 6 or 9 MU of recombinant interferon-α2a (Roferon-A, Hoffman-La Roche, Tokyo, Japan, or Canferon A, Takeda Pharmaceutical, Osaka, Japan) intramuscularly every day for the first 2 weeks and then three times a week for the following 22 weeks [13]. Another group of 132 cases was randomly assigned to receive either 6 or 10 MU of recombinant interferon-α2b (Intron A, Schering-Plough or Yamanouchi Pharmaceutical, Tokyo, Japan) intramuscularly every day for the first 2 weeks and then three times a week for the following 22 weeks [14]. A third group of 132 patients was treated with 6 MU of natural interferon-β (Toray Industries or Daiichi Pharmaceutical, Tokyo, Japan) by intravenous injection ranging from 252 to 264 MU [15]. This total amount of interferon-β is the ordinary dosage for treatment of chronic hepatitis C patients in Japan. A fourth group of 56 patients received 28-week or 52-week courses of natural interferon-α [11,16]. Five MU of natural interferon-α (Otsuka Pharmaceutical, Tokyo, Japan) was administered intramuscularly three times a week during the first 28 weeks. In the 52-week course, 5 MU of natural interferon-α was further administered twice a week during the following 24 weeks. A fifth group of 543 patients received 6 MU of natural interferon-α (human lymphoblastoid interferon, Sumitomo Pharmaceutical, Osaka, Japan) intramuscularly every day for the first 2 weeks and then three times a week for 14 or 22 weeks [10]. Retreatment with a 24-week course of natural interferon-α was done for 161 cases. Interferon treatment was given once for 861 cases, twice for 128 cases, three times for 23 cases, four times for eight cases, five times for one case, and six times for one case. After written informed consent had been obtained, clinical evaluation and laboratory tests including α-fetoprotein determination were performed before treatment, weekly during the first 2 weeks of treatment, biweekly for the remainder of the treatment, and monthly after the treatment, in order to classify the ALT response to interferon therapy.

Patients treated with interferon were divided into the following three groups, based on the change in serum ALT levels as described previously [10,11]. The first was the sustained-response group in which ALT levels remained within the normal range for more than 24 weeks after therapy. The second was the transient-response group in which ALT levels decreased to the normal range during therapy but then increased to abnormal levels in the following 24 weeks. The third was the no-response group in which ALT levels did not decrease during therapy or fluctuated.

Ultrasonography was carried out before interferon therapy and every 3–6 months after it. Before interferon therapy, none of the patients had HCC or suspicious space-occupying lesions as judged by ultrasonography or computed tomography. All 1022 cases were followed by both biochemical examinations including α-fetoprotein and ultrasonography. This study protocol was in accord with the Helsinki Declaration of 1975 (revision of 1983) and approved by the Ethical Committee of Osaka University School of Medicine.

Determination of HCV Genome Subtype

HCV was classified by either Okamoto's method [17] or Kohara's method [18]. In this study, HCV genome subtype 1a or 1b determined by the group-specific polymerase chain reaction [17] or serological genotype I determined by the enzyme-linked immunosorbent assay [18] was classified as subtype 1, while HCV genome subtypes 2a or 2b or serological genotype II was classified as subtype 2.

Determination of HCV RNA Levels

Serum HCV RNA levels were quantified using branched DNA (bDNA) probe assay (version 1; Chiron, Dai-ichi Kagaku, Tokyo) [16,19], competitive reverse transcription–polymerase chain reaction (RT-PCR) [10], or combined RT-PCR assay (Amplicor-HCV monitor assay) [20]. HCV RNA level of 10^5 copies/ml by the Amplicor-HCV monitor assay was already demonstrated to correspond to approximately 10^6 equivalents/ml by the bDNA probe assay [20]. Therefore, when the serum HCV RNA level was more than 10^6 equivalents/ml by bDNA assay, more than 10^6 copies/ml serum by competitive RT-PCR, or more than 10^5 copies/ml serum by Amplicor-HCV monitor assay, it was designated as a high viral load as described previously [10,16,20].

Histological Evaluation

Liver biopsy was carried out before interferon therapy in all cases. Specimens were fixed in formaldehyde and embedded in paraffin. The sections were stained with hematoxylin–eosin and Azan-Mallory, and analyzed by two pathologists without any knowledge of the clinical and laboratory data. Histological findings were scored according to the histological activity index (HAI) of Knodell et al. [21]. Thirty-four patients were histologically proven to have liver cirrhosis.

Diagnosis of Hepatocellular Carcinoma

Space-occupying lesions detected or suspected at the time of ultrasonography were further examined with computed tomography, selective hepatic angiography and fine-needle aspiration biopsy, unless the ultrasonographic findings confirmed that the lesions were unquestionably benign (e.g., hemangioma or cysts). A final diagnosis of

HCC was based on histological findings from resected hepatic tumors or biopsy specimens, or on the radiological findings of selective hepatic angiography.

Statistical Analysis

Age, histological scores before interferon therapy, total dosage of interferon, and period of observation are expressed as mean ± SD. The chi-squared test was used for statistical analysis of the comparison between group frequencies. When appropriate, the clinical and laboratory features of the two groups were compared by Student's t-test and Welch's test. As for comparison among the three groups, one-way analysis of variance was used. When data were not normally distributed, the Wilcoxon rank-sum test and Kruskal-Wallis test were used.

Independent factors associated with the development of HCC were studied with stepwise Cox regression analysis. Possible risk factors for the development of HCC included 13 variables: age; gender; total histological score; Knodell's scores for periportal necrosis, intralobular inflammation, portal inflammation, and fibrosis; classification of HCV subtype; pretreatment level of viremia; total dosage of administered interferon; number of times of interferon treatment; period of observation; and ALT response to interferon therapy. Each variable was transformed into the categorical data consisting of two or three simple ordinal numbers for multivariate analysis. All factors found to be at least marginally associated with carcinogenesis ($P < 0.15$) were tested by the multivariate Cox proportional hazard model. In addition, the same analysis was performed when histological diagnosis (chronic hepatitis or liver cirrhosis) was substituted as a variable for Knodell's histological scores themselves. The period of observation used in calculating the risk of HCC began at the end of the final interferon treatment and ended on the date of HCC diagnosis, the date of final ultrasonography, or the date of death, whichever came first. The method of Kaplan and Meier was used to estimate the cumulative risk of HCC, and the statistical significance of differences in this incidence was found by the generalized Wilcoxon signed-rank test.

Data analysis was performed with the SAS/PC statistical package (SAS Institute, Cary, NC, USA). All reported P-values were two-sided and a P-value of less than 0.05 was considered to be significant.

Results

Clinical Characteristics Before Interferon Therapy

A sustained response was observed in 313 cases, a transient response in 304 cases, and no response in 405 cases. There were no significant differences in age, gender, scores for intralobular inflammation and portal inflammation, and the total amount of administered interferon among the three groups. The total score of the histological activity index and scores for periportal necrosis and fibrosis were significantly higher in nonresponders than in sustained responders and transient responders ($P < 0.02$, $P < 0.02$, and $P < 0.0001$, respectively). According to the fibrosis score of the histological activity index, 5 (1.6%) of the sustained responders, 6 (2.0%) of the transient responders, and 23 (5.7%) of the nonresponders were diagnosed as having liver cirrhosis, with the frequency being significantly higher in nonresponders ($P < 0.01$). The rate of patients with a low viral load and the prevalence of HCV subtype 2 were significantly higher in sustained responders than in transient responders and nonresponders ($P < 0.0001$). The average period of observation was 38.9 ± 13.8 months (range 13 to 95 months) for sustained responders, 36.6 ± 11.3 months (range 13 to 85 months) for transient responders, and 36.9 ± 13.3 months (range 13 to 97 months) for nonresponders, with no significant difference among the three groups (Table 1).

Development of Hepatocellular Carcinoma

Forty-eight patients had a suspicious lesion of HCC as judged by ultrasonography and computed tomography. All 48 underwent angiography. A liver biopsy was done if indicated when the patients did not show typical tumor staining in the liver by angiography or were not diagnosed as having a particular disease, such as hemangioma. One patient was diagnosed as having cavernous hemangioma and another as having adenomatous hyperplasia by histological examination. A final diagnosis of HCC was made in 46 cases: 5 male sustained responders (serum HCV RNA was undetectable in all sustained responders at the time of HCC diagnosis), 9 male transient responders, and 32 (25 males and 7 females) nonresponders. Only 3 of 34 patients diagnosed as having liver cirrhosis before interferon therapy developed HCC, all of whom

Table 1. Clinical characteristics before interferon therapy according to alanine aminotransferase (ALT) responses to interferon in chronic hepatitis C (HCV) patients

Characteristic	Sustained response ($n = 313$)	Transient response ($n = 304$)	No response ($n = 405$)
Age (years)	52.4 ± 11.0	52.6 ± 9.9	53.5 ± 9.4
Male/female	211/102	202/102	275/130
HCV RNA level			
High viral load	55[a]	133	180
Low viral load	146[a]	74	80
N.T.	112	97	145
HCV subtype			
Group 1	111[a]	208	275
Group 2	109[a]	32	39
Mixed	8	3	0
Unclassified	3	0	1
N.T.	82	61	90
Total HAI score	9.0 ± 3.4	8.9 ± 3.6	9.6 ± 3.6[b]
Periportal necrosis	2.3 ± 1.7	2.3 ± 1.7	2.7 ± 1.8[b]
Intralobular inflammation	2.1 ± 1.1	2.0 ± 1.2	2.1 ± 1.1
Portal inflammation	2.6 ± 0.9	2.6 ± 0.9	2.6 ± 0.9
Fibrosis	1.9 ± 1.1	2.1 ± 1.0	2.3 ± 1.1[c]
Total dose of IFN (million units)	489 ± 195	497 ± 195	505 ± 338
Period of observation (months)	38.9 ± 13.8 (13–95)	36.6 ± 11.3 (13–85)	36.9 ± 13.3 (13–97)

N.T., not tested; HAI, histological activity index; IFN, interferon.
[a] $P < 0.0001$ vs transient response and no response; [b] $P < 0.02$ vs sustained response and transient response; [c] $P < 0.0001$ vs sustained response and transient response. (From [22] with permission)

were nonresponders. The average period from the completion of interferon therapy to the detection of HCC was 35 ± 13 months (range 21 to 54 months) for sustained responders, 28 ± 9 months (range 15 to 44 months) for transient responders, and 33 ± 13 months (range 14 to 70 months) for nonresponders, with no significant differences among the three groups.

Cumulative Risk of Hepatocellular Carcinoma

Figure 1 shows the Kaplan-Meier estimates of the cumulative risk of HCC, according to the ALT responses to interferon therapy. The cumulative incidence of HCC in transient responders was almost equal to that in

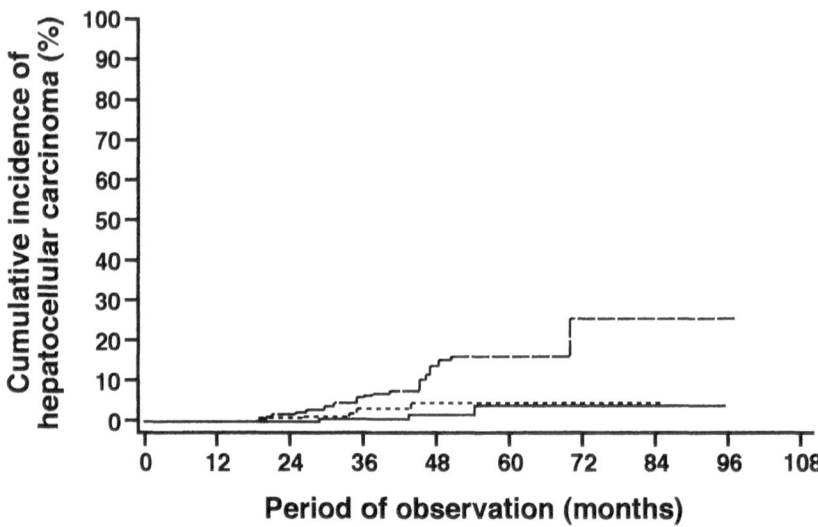

Fig. 1. Cumulative incidence of hepatocellular carcinoma in chronic hepatitis C patients according to ALT responses to interferon therapy. *Solid line,* sustained responders; *dotted line,* transient responders; *dashed line,* nonresponders (From [22] with permission)

sustained responders, and it was significantly higher in nonresponders than in sustained and transient responders (P = 0.0009). Whether the HCV classification was subtype 1 or 2, the cumulative incidence of HCC in nonresponders gradually rose and was significantly higher than in sustained and transient responders (P = 0.02 in HCV subtype 1, P = 0.01 in HCV subtype 2). There was no significant difference in the cumulative incidence of HCC between patients with HCV subtypes 1 and 2 (P = 0.14). Patients with advanced liver fibrosis (Knodell's fibrosis score $\geqq$3) showed a significantly higher cumulative incidence of HCC than those with mild fibrosis (fibrosis score $\leqq$1) (P = 0.0008). Males had a significantly higher cumulative incidence of HCC than females (P = 0.02). The older the patient was, the higher was the cumulative incidence of HCC (P = 0.002).

From the curves of the estimated cumulative incidence, the third-year appearance rates of HCC in sustained responders, transient responders and non-responders were predicted to be 1.6%, 3.4%, and 6.3%, the fifth-year rates to be 4.3%, 4.7%, and 21.4%, and the seventh-year rates to be 4.3%, 4.7%, and 26.1%, respectively.

Table 2. Risk factors responsible for the development of hepatocellular carcinoma after interferon treatment

Variable	Risk ratio	95% CI	P-Value
Age (years)			
<55	1.0		
≥55	4.65	1.56–13.84	0.006
Response to interferon			
Sustained response	1.0		
No response	7.90	1.74–35.93	0.008
Sustained response	1.0		
Transient response	3.12	0.59–16.60	0.18
Gender			
Female	1.0		
Male	4.35	1.26–14.96	0.02
Lobular inflammation			
≤1	1.0		
≥3	0.41	0.17–0.96	0.04
HCV RNA level			
Low viral load	1.0		
High viral load	2.35	1.02–5.43	0.045
Fibrosis			
≤1	1.0		
≥3	3.16	0.99–10.06	0.052

CI, confidence interval. (From [22] with permission)

Risk Factors for Hepatocellular Carcinoma

Cox proportional-hazards analysis was performed with the 13 variables mentioned above. Age, ALT response to interferon, gender, the degree of portal inflammation, and HCV RNA level were extracted as independent significant risk factors in the development of HCC and were adjusted simultaneously to estimate hazard rate ratios for the development of HCC (Table 2). When the patients were divided into two age groups, <55 and ≧55 years, those over 55 years had a significantly higher risk ratio (risk ratio, 4.65; 95% confidence interval (CI), 1.56–13.84) than those under 55 years ($P = 0.006$). A positive association was observed between the risk of HCC and ALT response to interferon therapy, demonstrating that the risk of HCC was 7.90-fold higher (95% CI, 1.74–35.93) for nonresponders than for sustained responders ($P = 0.008$). However, the risk of HCC was not elevated in transient responders, compared to sustained responders (risk ratio, 3.12; 95% CI, 0.59–16.60; $P = 0.18$). The risk of HCC in men was 4.35-times higher (95% CI, 1.26–14.96) than in women ($P = 0.02$). Portal inflammation was negatively associated with the appearance of HCC (risk ratio, 0.41; 95% CI, 0.17–0.96; $P = 0.04$), whereas the degree of fibrosis did not influence the appearance of HCC (risk ratio, 3.16; 95% CI, 0.99–10.06; $P = 0.052$). Patients with a high viral load had a significantly higher risk ratio (risk ratio, 2.35; 95% CI, 1.02–5.43; $P = 0.045$) than those with a low viral load. The presence of liver cirrhosis was not an independent risk factor for the development of HCC.

Discussion

HCV multiplication is sustained throughout the course of infection [23]. When hepatocytes are continuously damaged and replicated, as in chronic hepatitis C, the frequencies of genetic alterations probably increase, leading to the development of HCC. Therefore, adequate treatment for HCV eradication at the stage of chronic hepatitis C is considered to be important for prevention of HCC, because cirrhosis reduces the rate of response to interferon [24,25]. More than 200 000 patients with chronic hepatitis C have been treated with interferon in Japan. Several investigators reported its usefulness for virological and biochemical long-term outcome. Moreover, this treatment has been shown to alleviate liver fibrosis in addition to necrosis and inflammation in patients with HCV eradication and/or ALT normalization [11,12]. In cirrhotic patients, a significant reduction in the incidence of HCC was reported in patients treated with interferon [25,26]. These results suggest that the use of interferon in the treatment of patients with chronic hepatitis C and compensated cirrhosis may be beneficial in preventing the development of HCC, with the benefits greatest for patients who respond to interferon by normalizing ALT or clearing HCV. However, there have been no studies describing the risk factors for the development of HCC and its incidence after interferon therapy in patients with chronic hepatitis C. Even if the follow-up after the completion of interferon therapy may not be long enough, the risk factors for the development of HCC and its incidence should be clarified, to be able to identify patients with a high risk of developing HCC after interferon therapy.

In our present study, as expected, sustained responders showed the lowest possibility of HCC development. However, five sustained responders with HCV eradication did develop HCC, indicating the need for careful follow-up using ultrasonography for at least 5 years after interferon therapy (the longest interval from the completion of interferon therapy to the detection of HCC in sustained responders was 54 months). Interestingly, patients showing transient response did not have an elevated risk of HCC in comparison with sustained responders, and the cumulative incidence of HCC in transient responders was almost equal to that in sustained responders. Thus, HCC was less likely to develop in patients in whom interferon was effective for normalizing ALT during the therapy, even when HCV was not eradicated, probably due to the alleviation of hepatocyte necrosis and liver fibrosis in such patients, as previously described [11,12]. This might reduce the incidence of genetic abnormalities accumulating during cell division, resulting in lowering the risk of HCC. However, the seventh-year cumulative appearance rates of clinically and ultrasonographically evident liver cirrhosis in sustained responders, transient responders, and nonresponders were estimated to be 16.3%, 34.9%, and 64.5%, respectively (not shown), suggesting that the evolution of the disease was observed more often in transient responders than in sustained responders. Consequently, the cumulative incidence of HCC may increase, displaying a hyperbolic curve, in transient responders in the near future. On the other hand, patients showing no response had a greatly increased risk of HCC, demonstrating that the risk of HCC was 7.90-fold higher in non-responders compared to sustained responders.

The presence of liver cirrhosis was reported to be associated with higher HCC incidence than chronic hepatitis or poor response to interferon [25]. In our present investigation, liver cirrhosis was more frequently observed in nonresponders than in sustained responders and transient responders. However, the presence of liver cirrhosis itself was not found to be a risk factor for HCC development. This result suggests that not the presence of liver cirrhosis, but no response to interferon therapy, is strongly associated with the appearance of HCC. Furthermore, the degree of fibrosis was not a significant risk factor but a relative risk factor for HCC development.

The third-year cumulative risk of HCC was shown to be 3.8% for patients with chronic hepatitis [27]. In patients with chronic hepatitis C, the cumulative HCC incidence was reported to gradually increase and to be threefold higher than in those with chronic hepatitis B [3]. In the retrospective follow-up study of European patients with compensated cirrhosis type C, the 5-year risk of HCC was reported to be 7% [5]. In Japan, the appearance rate of HCC in cirrhotic patients with anti-HCV was reported to be 5%–7% per year [4,6]. In our present study, non-responders showed a significantly higher cumulative incidence of HCC than transient responders and sustained responders, regardless of HCV subtype. The probable appearance rate of HCC at the seventh year after interferon therapy was estimated to be 26.1% (approximately 3.7% per year). This incidence of HCC in nonresponders was almost equal to that of the natural course of chronic hepatitis C patients [3]. Unfortunately, almost all patients with chronic hepatitis C in Japan have been treated with interferon, except for cases with refusal of treatment, a history of psychiatric problems, the presence of decompensated liver cirrhosis, or autoimmune disease. Although there was a small number of patients with less active or a milder form of chronic hepatitis, they were judged to be inappropriate as controls. Therefore, we could not compare the risk ratio and the HCC incidence of nonresponders with those of chronic hepatitis C patients without interferon treatment. Although our results might be difficult to interpret due to the study being a nonrandomized one, we surmise that interferon therapy did not seem to prevent HCC in patients showing no response. Whether interferon can prevent liver carcinogenesis, especially in nonresponders, needs to be determined with future randomized controlled studies.

We would like to emphasize that the risk of HCC development is significantly low in chronic hepatitis C patients, for whom interferon is effective for normalizing ALT, even when HCV is not eradicated. This suggests that the aim of interferon therapy for chronic hepatitis C should be not only HCV eradication but also ALT normalization during interferon therapy, even if HCV is not eradicated, in order to reduce the incidence of HCC. Finally, we concluded that patients in the high-risk group of HCC after interferon therapy were those showing no response, who were older, and who were male, and that such patients should be carefully followed, using ultrasonography to detect HCC as early as possible.

Acknowledgments. In addition to the study authors, the following institutions and physicians were participants in the Osaka Liver Disease Study Group: Osaka National Hospital, M. Masuzawa and M. Kato; Osaka Rousai Hospital, H. Yoshihara and K. Suzuki; Osaka Kouseinenkin Hospital, T. Kashiwagi and M. Naito; The Center for Adult Disease Osaka, A. Inoue and T. Matsunaga; National Osaka South Hospital, T. Mukuda

and T. Hijioka; Higashiosaka City Central Hospital, H. Fusamoto and
H. Hagiwara; Kaizuka Municipal Hospital, S. Ooarai; Kansai Rousai Hos-
pital, S. Kashio; Nagahori Hospital, A. Terada; Osaka Kaisei Hospital, H.
Meren; Osaka Police Hospital, A. Asai; Osaka Prefectural Hospital,
T. Miyamoto; Shinsenri Hospital, T. Akeyama and M. Kono; and Yao
Municipal Hospital, H. Fukui. We thank Mr K. Nukui very much for the
statistical analysis.

References

1. DiBisceglie AM, Goodman ZD, Ishak KG, Hoofnagle JH, Melpolder JJ, Alter HJ
   (1991) Long-term clinical and histological follow-up of chronic posttransfusion
   hepatitis. Hepatology 14:969–974
2. Kiyosawa K, Sodeyama T, Tanaka E, Gibo Y, Yoshizawa K, Nagano Y, Furuta S,
   et al (1990) Interrelationship of blood transfusion, non-A, non-B hepatitis and
   hepatocellular carcinoma. Analysis by detection of antibody to hepatitis C virus.
   Hepatology 12:671–675
3. Takano S, Yokosuka O, Imazeki F, Tagawa M, Omata M (1995) Incidence of
   hepatocellular carcinoma in chronic hepatitis B and C. A prospective study of 251
   patients. Hepatology 21:650–655
4. Ikeda K, Saitoh S, Koida I, Arase Y, Tsubota A, Chayama K, Kumada H, et al
   (1993) A multivariate analysis of risk factors for hepatocellular carcinogenesis:
   a prospective observation of 795 patients with viral and alcoholic cirrhosis.
   Hepatology 18:47–53
5. Fattovich G, Giustina G, Degos F, Tremolada F, Diodati G, Almasio P, Nevens
   F, et al (1997) Morbidity and mortality in compensated cirrhosis type C:
   a retrospective follow-up study of 384 patients. Gastroenterology 112:463–
   472
6. Oka H, Kurioka N, Kim K, Kanno T, Kuroki T, Mizoguchi Y, Kobayashi K (1990)
   Prospective study of early detection of hepatocellular carcinoma in patients with
   cirrhosis. Hepatology 12:680–687
7. Davis GL, Balart LA, Schiff ER, Lindsay K, Bodenheimer HC, Rerrilo RP, Carey W,
   et al (1989) Treatment of chronic hepatitis C with recombinant interferon alpha.
   A multicenter randomized controlled trial. N Engl J Med 321:1501–1506
8. Di Bisceglie AM, Martin P, Kassianides C, Lisker-Melman M, Murray L, Waggoner
   J, Goodman Z, et al (1989) Recombinant interferon alpha therapy for chronic
   hepatitis C. A randomized, double blind placebo-controlled trial. N Engl J Med
   321:1506–1510
9. Hagiwara H, Hayashi N, Mita E, Ueda K, Takehara T, Kasahara A, Fusamoto H,
   et al (1992) Detection of hepatitis C virus RNA in serum of patients with chronic
   hepatitis C treated with interferon-α. Hepatology 15:37–41
10. Hagiwara H, Hayashi N, Mita E, Takehara T, Kasahara A, Fusamoto H, Kamada T
    (1993) Quantitative analysis of hepatitis C virus RNA in serum during interferon
    alfa therapy. Gastroenterology 104:877–883

11. Kasahara A, Hayashi N, Hiramatsu N, Oshita M, Hagiwara H, Katayama K, Kato M, et al (1995) Ability of prolonged interferon treatment to suppress relapse after cessation of therapy in patients with chronic hepatitis C: a multicenter randomized controlled trial. Hepatology 21:291-297

12. Hiramatsu N, Hayashi N, Kasahara A, Hagiwara H, Takehara T, Haruna Y, Naito M, et al (1995) Improvement of liver fibrosis in chronic hepatitis C patients treated with natural interferon alpha. J Hepatol 22:135-142

13. Hagiwara H, Hayashi N, Kasahara A, Oshita M, Katayama K, Kato M, Masuzawa M, et al (1996) Treatment with recombinant interferon-α 2a for patients with chronic hepatitis C: predictive factors for biochemical and virologic response. Scand J Gastroenterol 31:1021-1026

14. Kuzushita N, Hayashi N, Katayama K, Kanto T, Oshita M, Hagiwara H, Kasahara A, et al (1997) High levels of serum interleukin-10 are associated with a poor response to interferon treatment in patients with chronic hepatitis C. Scand J Gastroenterol 32:169-174

15. Kasahara A, Hayashi N, Mochizuki K, Oshita M, Katayama K, Kato M, Masuzawa M, et al (1997) Circulating matrix metalloproteinase-2 and tissue inhibitor of metalloproteinase-1 as serum markers of fibrosis in patients with chronic hepatitis C. Relationship to interferon response. J Hepatol 26:574-583

16. Yuki N, Hayashi N, Kasahara A, Hagiwara H, Takehara T, Oshita M, Katayama K, et al (1995) Pretreatment viral load and response to prolonged interferon-α course for chronic hepatitis C. J Hepatol 22:457-463

17. Okamoto H, Sugiyama Y, Okada S, Kurai K, Akahane Y, Sugai Y, Tanaka T, et al (1992) Typing hepatitis C virus by polymerase chain reaction with type-specific primers: application to clinical surveys and tracing infectious sources. J Gen Virol 73:673-679

18. Tanaka T, Tsukiyama-Kohara K, Yamaguchi K, Yagi S, Tanaka S, Hasegawa A, Ohta N, et al (1994) Significance of specific antibody assay for genotyping of hepatitis C virus. Hepatology 19:1347-1353

19. Lau YN, Davis G, Kniffen J, Qian K-P, Urdea MS, Chan CS, Mizokami M, et al (1993) Significance of serum hepatitis C virus RNA levels in chronic hepatitis C. Lancet 341:1501-1504

20. Shiratori Y, Kato N, Yokosuka O, Imazeki F, Hashimoto E, Hayashi N, Nakamura A, et al (1997) Predictors of the efficacy of interferon therapy in chronic hepatitis C virus infection. Gastroenterology 113:558-566

21. Knodell RG, Ishak KG, Black WC, Chen TS, Craig R, Kaplowitz N, Kiernan TW, et al (1981) Formulation and application of a numerical scoring system for assessing histological activity in asymptomatic chronic active hepatitis. Hepatology 1:431-435

22. Kasahara A, Hayashi N, Mochizuki K, et al. (1998) Risk factors for hepatocellular carcinoma and its incidence after interferon treatment in patients with chronic Hepatitis C. Hepatology 27:1394-1402

23. Hagiwara H, Hayashi N, Mita E, Naito M, Kasahara A, Fusamoto H, Kamada T (1993) Quantitation of hepatitis C virus RNA in serum of asymptomatic blood donors and patients with type C chronic liver disease. Hepatology 17:545-550

24. Jouet P, Roudot-Thoraval F, Dhumeaux D, Metreau JM (1994) Comparative efficacy of interferon alpha in cirrhotic and noncirrhotic patients with non-A, non-B, C hepatitis. Gastroenterology 106:686–690
25. Nishiguchi S, Kuroki T, Nakatani S, Morimoto H, Takeda T, Nakajima S, Shiomi S, et al (1995) Randomized trial of effects of interferon-α on incidence of hepatocellular carcinoma in chronic active hepatitis C with cirrhosis. Lancet 346:1051–1055
26. Mazzelia G, Accogli E, Sottili S, Festi G, Orsini M, Salzetta A, Novelli V, et al (1996) Alpha-interferon treatment may prevent hepatocellular carcinoma in HCV-related liver cirrhosis. J Hepatol 24:141–147
27. Tsukuma H, Hiyama T, Tanaka S, Nakao M, Yabuuchi T, Kitamura T, Nakanishi K, et al (1993) Risk factors for hepatocellular carcinoma among patients with chronic liver disease. N Engl J Med 328:1797–1801

Index